BOOST YOUR BRAIN COOKBOOK

Nourish Your Mind, Enhance Your Cognitive Power: A Delicious Guide to Boosting Brain Health Through Culinary Delights

ERIN P. WALKER

Table Of Contents

Introduction

Have you ever wondered if the food you eat could actually boost your brainpower? Can the meals we enjoy on a daily basis have a profound impact on our cognitive abilities, memory, and overall mental well-being? The answer, my friends, is a resounding yes!

Welcome to the "Boost Your Brain Cookbook," where we embark on a culinary journey to nourish our minds and enhance our cognitive power through the power of food. In this book, we will explore the fascinating science behind the link between nutrition and brain health, while providing you with a delectable array of recipes that are specifically designed to maximise your mental potential.

As we delve into this topic, let us pause and reflect on a few critical questions. How often do we consider the impact of our dietary choices on our brain? Do we truly understand the nutrients our brains need to function optimally? Are we actively seeking out ingredients and recipes that can enhance our cognitive function and promote mental clarity?

It's no secret that our brains are the epicentre of our existence, controlling every thought, emotion, and action. Yet, all too often, we neglect to prioritise its well-being when it comes to our diet. We meticulously plan our meals for weight loss, muscle gain, or heart health, but rarely do we consider the profound effects our choices have on our brain.

The truth is, the brain requires a delicate balance of essential nutrients to perform at its best. From omega-3 fatty acids and antioxidants to vitamins and minerals, each component plays a crucial role in supporting cognitive function, protecting against age-related decline, and even boosting our ability to learn and retain information.

So, how do we harness the power of food to unlock our brain's full potential? How can we transform our everyday meals into brain-boosting feasts? That's where this cookbook comes in. Within these pages, you will discover a wide range of mouthwatering recipes that are carefully crafted to nourish your mind and enhance your cognitive abilities.

From breakfast to dinner, snacks to desserts, and even beverages, every recipe has been meticulously designed to incorporate ingredients that are known to have a positive impact on brain health. Imagine starting your day with a creamy smoothie bowl packed with antioxidants and brain-boosting fruits, or savouring a delicious plant-based lunch that fuels your mind with essential nutrients.

But this book isn't just about providing you with delectable recipes. It's about empowering you with knowledge and understanding. Throughout the chapters, we will delve into the science behind brain-boosting foods, exploring the specific nutrients and compounds that contribute to enhanced cognitive function. We will also address critical questions such as: How do certain foods protect against age-related cognitive decline? Can nutrition impact our mood and mental well-being? And what role does mindful eating play in optimising brain health?

Additionally, we will guide you through meal planning tips and grocery shopping strategies to help you incorporate brain-healthy ingredients into your daily routine. We want to ensure that you not only enjoy the recipes in this book but also develop a sustainable and nourishing approach to fueling your mind for years to come.

So, are you ready to embark on this culinary adventure that will not only tantalise your taste buds but also sharpen your mind? Are you ready to explore the incredible potential of food to enhance your cognitive abilities, memory, and overall mental wellness? If the answer is a resounding yes, then let's dive into the "Boost Your Brain Cookbook" and unlock the secrets to a sharper, more vibrant brain.

Chapter 1: The Science of Brain-Boosting Foods

In our modern, fast-paced lives, we often find ourselves searching for ways to optimise our cognitive abilities and enhance our mental well-being. While there are numerous strategies and techniques available, one often overlooked aspect is the impact of our diet on brain health. The science of brain-boosting foods reveals that what we eat can significantly influence our cognitive function, memory, and overall brain health.

Research has shown that certain nutrients and bioactive compounds found in foods can have a profound impact on the structure and function of our brains. These brain-boosting foods are often rich in antioxidants, healthy fats, vitamins, minerals, and phytochemicals, all of which play essential roles in supporting optimal brain function.

One key group of brain-boosting nutrients is omega-3 fatty acids, particularly docosahexaenoic acid (DHA). DHA is a crucial component of brain cell membranes and is believed to contribute to improved cognitive function and enhanced memory. Fatty fish, such as salmon, mackerel, and sardines, are excellent sources of DHA. Additionally, plant-based sources like chia seeds, flaxseeds, and walnuts provide alpha-linolenic acid (ALA), which can be converted to DHA in the body.

Antioxidants, another vital group of compounds, play a crucial role in protecting the brain from oxidative stress and inflammation. Oxidative stress can lead to damage and deterioration of brain cells over time. Foods rich in antioxidants, such as berries, dark chocolate, green leafy vegetables, and colourful fruits, can help combat oxidative stress and promote brain health.

Moreover, B vitamins, including folate, vitamin B6, and vitamin B12, are essential for brain health. These vitamins play a vital role in the production of neurotransmitters, which are chemical messengers that facilitate communication between brain cells. Leafy greens, legumes, whole grains, and animal products like eggs and dairy are excellent sources of B vitamins.

Curcumin, a compound found in turmeric, has gained significant attention for its potential brain-boosting properties. Curcumin exhibits potent anti-inflammatory and antioxidant effects, which can help protect the brain from age-related decline and improve cognitive function. Incorporating turmeric into meals or consuming it as a supplement may have potential benefits for brain health.

Furthermore, polyphenols, a diverse group of compounds found in plants, have shown promising effects on brain health. These compounds possess antioxidant and anti-inflammatory properties and may help improve memory and cognitive function. Foods rich in polyphenols include green tea, dark chocolate, berries, and colourful vegetables.

The gut-brain connection is another fascinating aspect of the science of brain-boosting foods. Emerging research suggests that the microbiota, the trillions of microorganisms residing in our gut, can influence brain health and cognitive function. Fermented foods like yoghurt, sauerkraut, and kimchi contain beneficial probiotics that support a healthy gut microbiota, which in turn may positively impact brain health.

It is important to note that while individual nutrients and compounds have been studied for their brain-boosting properties, the overall dietary pattern is equally crucial. Following a balanced diet that includes a variety of nutrient-dense foods is key to supporting overall brain health.

In conclusion, the science of brain-boosting foods highlights the profound impact our diet can have on cognitive function and brain health. Nutrients like omega-3 fatty acids, antioxidants, B vitamins, curcumin, polyphenols, and a healthy gut microbiota all contribute to optimising brain function and protecting against age-related decline. By incorporating these brain-boosting foods into our daily meals, we can nourish our minds, enhance our cognitive abilities, and promote long-term brain health.

Understanding the Link Between Nutrition and Cognitive Function

The connection between nutrition and cognitive function has become an increasingly important area of study in recent years. Research has shown that the foods we consume play a significant role in shaping our brain health and cognitive abilities. By understanding this link, we can make informed dietary choices that support optimal cognitive function and overall brain health.

One of the key ways nutrition impacts cognitive function is through the supply of essential nutrients that our brain requires to function properly. These nutrients include vitamins, minerals, antioxidants, healthy fats, and amino acids. Each of these components plays a specific role in supporting brain health and cognitive processes.

For example, vitamins such as vitamin B12, folate, and vitamin E are essential for the production and maintenance of brain cells and neurotransmitters. These neurotransmitters, such as serotonin and dopamine, are crucial for regulating mood, memory, and overall cognitive function.

Minerals like iron, zinc, and magnesium are also vital for brain health. Iron is necessary for the delivery of oxygen to the brain, while zinc and magnesium play roles in neurotransmitter function and synaptic plasticity, which is the brain's ability to form and strengthen neural connections.

Antioxidants, such as vitamin C, vitamin E, and polyphenols, protect the brain from oxidative stress and inflammation. Oxidative stress can damage brain cells and contribute to age-related cognitive decline. By consuming foods rich in antioxidants, we can help mitigate this damage and support brain health.

Healthy fats, particularly omega-3 fatty acids, are crucial for brain function. The brain is composed of nearly 60% fat, and omega-3 fatty acids, specifically docosahexaenoic acid (DHA), are essential for maintaining brain cell structure and facilitating communication between neurons. Consuming foods rich in omega-3 fatty acids, such as fatty fish, flaxseeds, and walnuts, can support cognitive function and may even help protect against cognitive decline.

Furthermore, the impact of nutrition on cognitive function extends beyond individual nutrients. Dietary patterns, such as the Mediterranean diet or the DASH (Dietary Approaches to Stop Hypertension) diet, have been associated with better cognitive function and a lower risk of cognitive decline. These dietary patterns emphasise whole foods, including fruits, vegetables, whole grains, lean proteins, and healthy fats, while minimising processed foods, added sugars, and unhealthy fats.

The gut-brain axis, a bidirectional communication system between the gut and the brain, also plays a significant role in cognitive function. The gut microbiota, the collection of microorganisms residing in our digestive system, can influence brain health and cognitive processes. A healthy gut microbiota is associated with improved cognitive function and a reduced risk of conditions such as depression and anxiety. Consuming a diet rich in fibre, prebiotics, and fermented foods can support a diverse and healthy gut microbiota, ultimately benefiting cognitive function.

It is important to note that nutrition is just one piece of the puzzle when it comes to cognitive function. Other lifestyle factors, such as physical activity, sleep, stress management, and social engagement, also contribute to brain health. However, nutrition provides a unique opportunity to directly support brain health and optimise cognitive function.

Understanding the link between nutrition and cognitive function is crucial for making informed dietary choices that support brain health. Essential nutrients, antioxidants, healthy fats, and a balanced diet all contribute to optimal cognitive function. By adopting a diet rich in nutrient-dense foods and promoting a healthy gut microbiota, we can nourish our brains, enhance cognitive abilities, and support long-term brain health.

Essential Nutrients for Optimal Brain Health

The brain is a complex organ that requires a wide range of nutrients to function optimally. These essential nutrients play crucial roles in supporting brain health, cognitive function, and overall mental well-being. By understanding the importance of these nutrients, we can make informed dietary choices that promote optimal brain health.

1. Omega-3 Fatty Acids: Omega-3 fatty acids, particularly docosahexaenoic acid (DHA), are essential for brain health. DHA is a major component of brain cell membranes and plays a crucial role in maintaining their integrity. It is involved in various brain functions, including neurotransmission, synaptic plasticity, and inflammation regulation. Fatty fish, such as salmon, mackerel, and sardines, are excellent sources of DHA. Plant-based sources, such as chia seeds, flaxseeds, and walnuts, provide alpha-linolenic acid (ALA), which can be converted to DHA in the body.

2. Antioxidants: The brain is highly susceptible to oxidative stress, which can lead to the accumulation of harmful free radicals and damage to brain cells. Antioxidants help neutralise these free radicals and protect the brain from oxidative damage. Vitamins C and E, along with polyphenols found in fruits,

vegetables, and dark chocolate, are powerful antioxidants that support brain health.

3. B Vitamins: B vitamins, including folate, vitamin B6, and vitamin B12, are essential for brain function. They play key roles in the production of neurotransmitters, such as serotonin, dopamine, and norepinephrine, which regulate mood, memory, and cognitive function. Leafy greens, legumes, whole grains, eggs, and lean meats are excellent sources of B vitamins.

4. Vitamin D: Vitamin D is not only important for bone health but also plays a role in brain health. Low levels of vitamin D have been associated with an increased risk of cognitive decline and neurodegenerative diseases. Sunlight exposure, fortified dairy products, fatty fish, and egg yolks are good sources of vitamin D.

5. Magnesium: Magnesium is involved in over 300 enzymatic reactions in the body, including those related to brain function. It plays a role in neurotransmitter release, synaptic plasticity, and overall brain health. Good sources of magnesium include leafy greens, nuts, seeds, and whole grains.

6. Zinc: Zinc is essential for cognitive function and memory formation. It is involved in the production and regulation of neurotransmitters, as well as maintaining the structural integrity of brain cells. Oysters, beef, poultry, legumes, and nuts are good sources of zinc.

7. Iron: Iron is necessary for oxygen transport to the brain and is involved in energy production and neurotransmitter synthesis. Iron deficiency can lead to cognitive impairment and poor cognitive development in children. Good sources of iron include lean meats, poultry, fish, legumes, and dark leafy greens.

8. Choline: Choline is a precursor to acetylcholine, a neurotransmitter involved in memory and cognitive function. It also plays a role in brain development and maintenance. Eggs, liver, soybeans, and cruciferous vegetables are good sources of choline.

9. Vitamin K: Vitamin K is important for brain health as it helps regulate calcium levels in the brain, which is crucial for neuronal function. Green leafy vegetables, broccoli, and Brussels sprouts are good sources of vitamin K.

10. Water: While not a nutrient per se, proper hydration is essential for optimal brain function. Dehydration can impair cognitive performance and lead to fatigue and brain fog. It is important to drink enough water throughout the day to maintain hydration.

A well-balanced diet that includes these essential nutrients is crucial for optimal brain health. Incorporating foods rich in omega-3 fatty acids, antioxidants, B vitamins, vitamin D, magnesium, zinc, iron, choline, vitamin K, and staying hydrated can support cognitive function, memory, and overall brain health. As always, it is important to consult with a healthcare professional or registered dietitian for personalised advice and guidance on dietary needs.

Chapter 2: Breakfast Recipes to Fuel Your Mind

1. Avocado Toast:

Ingredients:

- 2 slices of whole grain bread

- 1 ripe avocado

- Salt and pepper to taste

- Optional toppings: sliced tomatoes, feta cheese, or a drizzle of olive oil

Instructions:

- Toast the bread until golden brown.

- Mash the avocado in a bowl and season with salt and pepper.

- Spread the mashed avocado on the toast.

- Add your desired toppings and enjoy!

2. Greek Yogurtparfait:

Ingredients:

- 1 cup Greek yoghourt

- 1/2 cup granola
- Fresh berries (strawberries, blueberries, raspberries)
- Honey or maple syrup for drizzling

Instructions:
- In a glass or bowl, layer Greek yoghurt, granola, and fresh berries.
- Repeat the layers until all ingredients are used.
- Drizzle with honey or maple syrup before serving.

3. Spinach and Mushroom Omelette:
Ingredients:
- 3 eggs
- Handful of spinach leaves
- 1/4 cup sliced mushrooms
- Salt and pepper to taste
- Grated cheese (optional)

Instructions:
- In a bowl, whisk the eggs until well beaten.

- Heat a non-stick pan over medium heat and add the spinach and mushrooms.
- Sauté until wilted and lightly browned.
- Pour the whisked eggs over the vegetables and season with salt and pepper.
- Cook until the omelette is set and lightly golden.
- Sprinkle with grated cheese if desired, fold in half, and serve.

4. Banana Pancakes:
Ingredients:
- 1 ripe banana, mashed
- 1 cup flour
- 1 cup milk
- 1 egg
- 1 tablespoon sugar
- 1 teaspoon baking powder
- Butter or oil for cooking

Instructions:

- In a bowl, combine mashed banana, flour, milk, egg, sugar, and baking powder.
- Stir until the batter is smooth.
- Heat a non-stick pan or griddle over medium heat and add butter or oil.
- Pour about 1/4 cup of batter onto the pan for each pancake.
- Cook until bubbles form on the surface, then flip and cook until golden brown.
- Serve with your favourite toppings, such as maple syrup or fresh fruit.

5. Chia Seed Pudding:
Ingredients:
- 1/4 cup chia seeds
- 1 cup milk (dairy or plant-based)
- 1 tablespoon honey or maple syrup
- Fresh fruit or nuts for topping

Instructions:

- In a jar or bowl, combine chia seeds, milk, and sweetener.

- Stir well to make sure the chia seeds are evenly distributed.

- Let it sit for 5 minutes, then stir again to prevent clumping.

- Cover and refrigerate overnight or for at least 2 hours.

- Top with fresh fruit or nuts before serving.

6. Veggie Breakfast Burrito:

Ingredients:

- 2 large tortillas
- 4 eggs, scrambled
- 1/2 cup diced bell peppers
- 1/2 cup diced onions
- 1/2 cup shredded cheese
- Salt and pepper to taste
- Salsa or avocado for serving

Instructions:

- In a pan, sauté the bell peppers and onions until softened.
- Add the scrambled eggs and cook until set.
- Season with salt and pepper.
- Warm the tortillas in a separate pan or microwave.
- Divide the egg mixture between the tortillas and top with shredded cheese.
- Roll up the tortillas, tucking in the sides, and serve with salsa or avocado.

7. Overnight Oats:
Ingredients:
- 1/2 cup rolled oats
- 1/2 cup milk (dairy or plant-based)
- 1/2 cup Greek yoghourt
- 1 tablespoon chia seeds
- 1 tablespoon honey or maple syrup
- Fresh fruit or nuts for topping

Instructions:

- In a jar or container, combine rolled oats, milk, Greek yoghurt, chia seeds, and sweetener.
- Stir well to combine.
- Cover and refrigerate overnight or for at least 4 hours.
- In the morning, give it a good stir and top with fresh fruit or nuts before serving.

8. Smashed Chickpea Toast:
Ingredients:
- 2 slices of whole grain bread
- 1/2 cup canned chickpeas, drained and rinsed
- 1 tablespoon lemon juice
- 1 tablespoon olive oil
- Salt and pepper to taste
- Optional toppings: sliced tomatoes, cucumber, or fresh herbs

Instructions:
- Toast the bread until golden brown.
- In a bowl, mash the chickpeas with a fork.

- Add lemon juice, olive oil, salt, and pepper to the mashed chickpeas and mix well.
- Spread the chickpea mixture on the toast.
- Add your desired toppings and enjoy!

9. Green Smoothie:

Ingredients:
- 1 cup spinach or kale
- 1 ripe banana
- 1/2 cup Greek yoghourt
- 1/2 cup milk (dairy or plant-based)
- 1 tablespoon honey or maple syrup
- Ice cubes (optional)

Instructions:
- In a blender, combine spinach or kale, banana, Greek yoghurt, milk, and sweetener.
- Blend until smooth and creamy.
- Add ice cubes if desired and blend again.
- Pour into a glass and enjoy!

10. Egg Muffins:
Ingredients:
- 6 eggs
- 1/2 cup diced vegetables (bell peppers, onions, spinach, etc.)
- 1/2 cup shredded cheese
- Salt and pepper to taste

Instructions:
- Preheat the oven to 350°F (175°C) and grease a muffin tin.
- In a bowl, whisk the eggs until well beaten.
- Stir in the diced vegetables, shredded cheese, salt, and pepper.
- Pour the egg mixture evenly into the muffin tin.
- Bake for 20-25 minutes or until the egg muffins are set and lightly golden.
- Allow them to cool slightly before removing from the tin.
- Serve warm or refrigerate for later use.

11. Quinoa Breakfast Bowl:

Ingredients:

- 1/2 cup cooked quinoa

- 1/2 cup Greek yoghourt

- Fresh berries

- Chopped nuts (almonds, walnuts, etc.)

- Honey or maple syrup for drizzling

Instructions:

- In a bowl, layer cooked quinoa, Greek yoghurt, fresh berries, and chopped nuts.

- Drizzle with honey or maple syrup before serving.

12. Peanut Butter Banana Smoothie:

Ingredients:

- 1 ripe banana

- 2 tablespoons peanut butter

- 1 cup milk (dairy or plant-based)

- 1 tablespoon honey or maple syrup

- Ice cubes (optional)

Instructions:
- In a blender, combine the ripe banana, peanut butter, milk, and sweetener.
- Blend until smooth and creamy.
- Add ice cubes if desired and blend again.
- Pour into a glass and enjoy!

13. Baked Egg Cups:
Ingredients:
- 6 slices of ham or turkey
- 6 eggs
- Salt and pepper to taste
- Optional toppings: shredded cheese, diced vegetables, or herbs

Instructions:
- Preheat the oven to 375°F (190°C) and grease a muffin tin.
- Place a slice of ham or turkey into each muffin cup, forming a cup shape.
- Crack an egg into each ham cup.

- Season with salt and pepper, and add desired toppings.
- Bake for 12-15 minutes or until the egg whites are set and the yolks are still slightly runny.
- Allow them to cool slightly before removing from the tin.
- Serve warm or refrigerate for later use.

14. Blueberry Quinoa Pancakes:
Ingredients:
- 1/2 cup cooked quinoa
- 1/2 cup flour
- 1/2 cup milk (dairy or plant-based)
- 1 egg
- 1 tablespoon sugar
- 1 teaspoon baking powder
- 1/2 cup fresh blueberries
- Butter or oil for cooking

Instructions:

- In a bowl, combine cooked quinoa, flour, milk, egg, sugar, and baking powder.
- Stir until the batter is smooth.
- Gently fold in the fresh blueberries.
- Heat a non-stick pan or griddle over medium heat and add butter or oil.
- Pour about 1/4 cup of batter onto the pan for each pancake.
- Cook until bubbles form on the surface, then flip and cook until golden brown.
- Serve with your favourite toppings, such as maple syrup or additional blueberries.

15. Breakfast Quesadilla:
Ingredients:
- 2 large tortillas
- 2 eggs, scrambled
- 1/2 cup shredded cheese
- 1/4 cup diced tomatoes
- 1/4 cup diced onions
- Salt and pepper to taste

- Salsa or avocado for serving

Instructions:

- Heat a non-stick pan over medium heat and add the scrambled eggs, shredded cheese, tomatoes, onions, salt, and pepper.
- Cook until the eggs are set and the cheese is melted.
- Warm the tortillas in a separate pan or microwave.
- Divide the egg mixture between the tortillas.
- Fold the tortillas in half and cook in a pan until lightly crispy on both sides.
- Serve with salsa or avocado.

Energising Smoothie Bowls

1. Berry Blast Bowl:

Ingredients:

- 1 cup mixed berries (strawberries, blueberries, raspberries)
- 1 frozen banana
- 1/2 cup almond milk

- 1 tablespoon chia seeds
- Toppings: granola, sliced almonds, fresh berries

Instructions:
1. Blend the mixed berries, frozen banana, almond milk, and chia seeds until smooth.
2. Pour the smoothie into a bowl.
3. Top with granola, sliced almonds, and fresh berries.

2. Green Goddess Bowl:
Ingredients:
- 2 cups spinach
- 1 frozen banana
- 1/2 cup pineapple chunks
- 1 tablespoon almond butter
- 1 cup coconut water
- Toppings: sliced kiwi, shredded coconut, hemp seeds

Instructions:

1. Blend the spinach, frozen banana, pineapple chunks, almond butter, and coconut water until smooth.

2. Pour the smoothie into a bowl.

3. Top with sliced kiwi, shredded coconut, and hemp seeds.

3. Chocolate Avocado Bowl:

Ingredients:

- 1 ripe avocado

- 2 tablespoons cocoa powder

- 1 frozen banana

- 1 cup almond milk

- 1 tablespoon honey or maple syrup

- Toppings: cacao nibs, sliced banana, chopped nuts

Instructions:

1. Blend the avocado, cocoa powder, frozen banana, almond milk, and sweetener until smooth.

2. Pour the smoothie into a bowl.

3. Top with cacao nibs, sliced banana, and chopped nuts.

4. Tropical Delight Bowl:
Ingredients:
- 1 cup frozen mango chunks
- 1/2 cup frozen pineapple chunks
- 1 frozen banana
- 1 cup coconut milk
- 1 tablespoon flaxseed meal
- Toppings: sliced mango, toasted coconut flakes, chia seeds

Instructions:
1. Blend the frozen mango chunks, frozen pineapple chunks, frozen banana, coconut milk, and flaxseed meal until smooth.
2. Pour the smoothie into a bowl.
3. Top with sliced mango, toasted coconut flakes, and chia seeds.

5. Peanut Butter Power Bowl:

Ingredients:

- 2 tablespoons peanut butter

- 1 frozen banana

- 1 cup almond milk

- 1 tablespoon honey or maple syrup

- 1/4 cup rolled oats

- Toppings: sliced banana, peanut butter drizzle, crushed peanuts

Instructions:

1. Blend the peanut butter, frozen banana, almond milk, honey or maple syrup, and rolled oats until smooth.

2. Pour the smoothie into a bowl.

3. Top with sliced banana, a drizzle of peanut butter, and crushed peanuts.

6. Acai Berry Bowl:

Ingredients:

- 1 packet frozen acai puree

- 1 frozen banana
- 1/2 cup mixed berries
- 1/2 cup almond milk
- 1 tablespoon honey or maple syrup
- Toppings: granola, sliced strawberries, chia seeds

Instructions:

1. Blend the frozen acai puree, frozen banana, mixed berries, almond milk, and honey or maple syrup until smooth.

2. Pour the smoothie into a bowl.

3. Top with granola, sliced strawberries, and chia seeds.

7. Matcha Green Tea Bowl:

Ingredients:

- 1 teaspoon matcha green tea powder
- 1 frozen banana
- 1 cup spinach
- 1 cup almond milk
- 1 tablespoon honey or maple syrup

- Toppings: sliced kiwi, coconut flakes, hemp seeds

Instructions:
1. Blend the matcha green tea powder, frozen banana, spinach, almond milk, and honey or maple syrup until smooth.
2. Pour the smoothie into a bowl.
3. Top with sliced kiwi, coconut flakes, and hemp seeds.

8. Blueberry Bliss Bowl:
Ingredients:
- 1 cup frozen blueberries
- 1 frozen banana
- 1/2 cup Greek yoghourt
- 1/2 cup almond milk
- 1 tablespoon honey or maple syrup
- Toppings: fresh blueberries, granola, sliced almonds

Instructions:

1. Blend the frozen blueberries, frozen banana, Greek yoghurt, almond milk, and honey or maple syrup until smooth.
2. Pour the smoothie into a bowl.
3. Top with fresh blueberries, granola, and sliced almonds.

9. Coconut Mango Bowl:
Ingredients:
- 1 cup frozen mango chunks
- 1/2 cup coconut milk
- 1/2 cup pineapple juice
- 1 tablespoon lime juice
- 1 tablespoon shredded coconut
- Toppings: sliced mango, toasted coconut flakes, mint leaves

Instructions:
1. Blend the frozen mango chunks, coconut milk, pineapple juice, lime juice, and shredded coconut until smooth.

2. Pour the smoothie into a bowl.

3. Top with sliced mango, toasted coconut flakes, and mint leaves.

10. Coffee Kick Bowl:

Ingredients:

- 1 cup cold brew coffee

- 1 frozen banana

- 1/2 cup almond milk

- 1 tablespoon almond butter

- 1 tablespoon honey or maple syrup

- Toppings: granola, cocoa powder, sliced almonds

Instructions:

1. Blend the cold brew coffee, frozen banana, almond milk, almond butter, and honey or maple syrup until smooth.

2. Pour the smoothie into a bowl.

3. Top with granola, cocoa powder, and sliced almonds.

Brain-Boosting Oatmeal Variations

1. Blueberry Walnut Oatmeal:

Ingredients:

- 1/2 cup rolled oats

- 1 cup almond milk

- 1/2 cup blueberries

- 2 tablespoons chopped walnuts

- 1 tablespoon honey or maple syrup

Instructions:

1. In a saucepan, combine the rolled oats and almond milk.

2. Cook over medium heat until the oats are creamy and tender.

3. Stir in the blueberries, walnuts, and sweetener.

4. Cook for another 2-3 minutes, until the blueberries are softened.

5. Serve hot.

2. Banana Almond Butter Oatmeal:

Ingredients:

- 1/2 cup rolled oats
- 1 cup almond milk
- 1 ripe banana, mashed
- 1 tablespoon almond butter
- 1 tablespoon honey or maple syrup

Instructions:
1. In a saucepan, combine the rolled oats and almond milk.
2. Cook over medium heat until the oats are creamy and tender.
3. Stir in the mashed banana, almond butter, and sweetener.
4. Cook for another 2-3 minutes, until well combined.
5. Serve hot.

3. Apple Cinnamon Oatmeal:
Ingredients:
- 1/2 cup rolled oats
- 1 cup water

- 1/2 cup diced apple
- 1/2 teaspoon cinnamon
- 1 tablespoon honey or maple syrup

Instructions:
1. In a saucepan, combine the rolled oats and water.
2. Cook over medium heat until the oats are creamy and tender.
3. Stir in the diced apple, cinnamon, and sweetener.
4. Cook for another 2-3 minutes, until the apple is softened.
5. Serve hot.

4. Matcha Green Tea Oatmeal:
Ingredients:
- 1/2 cup rolled oats
- 1 cup almond milk
- 1 teaspoon matcha green tea powder
- 1 tablespoon honey or maple syrup
- Toppings: sliced banana, chia seeds, shredded coconut

Instructions:

1. In a saucepan, combine the rolled oats and almond milk.

2. Cook over medium heat until the oats are creamy and tender.

3. Stir in the matcha green tea powder and sweetener.

4. Cook for another 2-3 minutes, until well combined.

5. Serve hot and top with sliced banana, chia seeds, and shredded coconut.

5. Peanut Butter Chocolate Chip Oatmeal:

Ingredients:

- 1/2 cup rolled oats

- 1 cup almond milk

- 1 tablespoon peanut butter

- 1 tablespoon cocoa powder

- 1 tablespoon honey or maple syrup

- 1 tablespoon chocolate chips

Instructions:

1. In a saucepan, combine the rolled oats and almond milk.

2. Cook over medium heat until the oats are creamy and tender.

3. Stir in the peanut butter, cocoa powder, and sweetener.

4. Cook for another 2-3 minutes, until well combined.

5. Serve hot and sprinkle with chocolate chips.

6. Mixed Berry Chia Oatmeal:

Ingredients:

- 1/2 cup rolled oats

- 1 cup almond milk

- 1/2 cup mixed berries (strawberries, blueberries, raspberries)

- 1 tablespoon chia seeds

- 1 tablespoon honey or maple syrup

Instructions:

1. In a saucepan, combine the rolled oats and almond milk.

2. Cook over medium heat until the oats are creamy and tender.

3. Stir in the mixed berries, chia seeds, and sweetener.

4. Cook for another 2-3 minutes, until the berries are softened.

5. Serve hot.

7. Coconut Mango Oatmeal:

Ingredients:

- 1/2 cup rolled oats

- 1 cup coconut milk

- 1/2 cup diced mango

- 1 tablespoon shredded coconut

- 1 tablespoon honey or maple syrup

Instructions:

1. In a saucepan, combine the rolled oats and coconut milk.

2. Cook over medium heat until the oats are creamy and tender.

3. Stir in the diced mango, shredded coconut, and sweetener.

4. Cook for another 2-3 minutes, until well combined.

5. Serve hot.

8. Turmeric Ginger Oatmeal:

Ingredients:

- 1/2 cup rolled oats

- 1 cup water

- 1/2 teaspoon ground turmeric

- 1/2 teaspoon grated ginger

- 1 tablespoon honey or maple syrup

- Toppings: sliced banana, chopped almonds, ground cinnamon

Instructions:

1. In a saucepan, combine the rolled oats and water.

2. Cook over medium heat until the oats are creamy and tender.

3. Stir in the ground turmeric, grated ginger, and sweetener.

4. Cook for another 2-3 minutes, until well combined.

5. Serve hot and top with sliced banana, chopped almonds, and ground cinnamon.

9. Pecan Maple Oatmeal:

Ingredients:

- 1/2 cup rolled oats

- 1 cup almond milk

- 2 tablespoons chopped pecans

- 1 tablespoon maple syrup

- 1/2 teaspoon vanilla extract

Instructions:

1. In a saucepan, combine the rolled oats and almond milk.

2. Cook over medium heat until the oats are creamy and tender.

3. Stir in the chopped pecans, maple syrup, and vanilla extract.

4. Cook for another 2-3 minutes, until well combined.

5. Serve hot.

10. Raspberry Dark Chocolate Oatmeal:

Ingredients:

- 1/2 cup rolled oats

- 1 cup water

- 1/2 cup fresh or frozen raspberries

- 1 tablespoon dark chocolate chips

- 1 tablespoon honey or maple syrup

Instructions:

1. In a saucepan, combine the rolled oats and water.

2. Cook over medium heat until the oats are creamy and tender.

3. Stir in the raspberries, dark chocolate chips, and sweetener.

4. Cook for another 2-3 minutes, until the raspberries are softened.

5. Serve hot.

Power-Packed Egg Dishes

1. Spinach and Mushroom Omelette:

Ingredients:

- 2 eggs
- 1/4 cup sliced mushrooms
- 1/4 cup fresh spinach leaves
- 2 tablespoons diced onions
- Salt and pepper to taste
- 1 tablespoon olive oil

Instructions:

1. In a bowl, whisk the eggs until well beaten. Season with salt and pepper.

2. Heat the olive oil in a skillet over medium heat.

3. Add the onions and mushrooms, and sauté until the mushrooms are tender.
4. Add the spinach leaves and cook for another minute until wilted.
5. Pour the beaten eggs into the skillet, spreading them evenly.
6. Cook until the edges start to set, then gently fold the omelette in half.
7. Cook for another minute until the eggs are cooked through.
8. Serve hot.

2. Smoked Salmon and Avocado Toast:
Ingredients:
- 2 slices of whole grain bread
- 2 hard-boiled eggs, sliced
- 2 ounces smoked salmon
- 1/2 avocado, sliced
- Fresh dill for garnish
- Salt and pepper to taste

Instructions:

1. Toast the slices of whole grain bread.

2. Spread the avocado slices on each slice of toast.

3. Layer the smoked salmon on top of the avocado.

4. Arrange the sliced hard-boiled eggs on top of the smoked salmon.

5. Season with salt and pepper, and garnish with fresh dill.

6. Serve immediately.

3. Spinach and Feta Breakfast Wrap:

Ingredients:

- 2 large eggs

- 1/4 cup fresh spinach leaves

- 2 tablespoons crumbled feta cheese

- 1 whole wheat tortilla

- Salt and pepper to taste

- 1 tablespoon olive oil

Instructions:

1. In a bowl, beat the eggs and season with salt and pepper.

2. Heat the olive oil in a skillet over medium heat.

3. Add the spinach leaves and sauté until wilted.

4. Pour the beaten eggs into the skillet, stirring gently until cooked through.

5. Sprinkle the crumbled feta cheese on top of the cooked eggs.

6. Warm the whole wheat tortilla in a separate skillet or microwave.

7. Spoon the egg mixture onto the tortilla and wrap it up.

8. Serve warm.

4. Veggie Egg Muffins:

Ingredients:

- 6 eggs
- 1/2 cup diced bell peppers (any colour)
- 1/2 cup diced zucchini
- 1/4 cup diced onions
- 1/4 cup shredded cheddar cheese

- Salt and pepper to taste
- Cooking spray

Instructions:
1. Preheat the oven to 350°F (175°C) and grease a muffin tin with cooking spray.
2. In a bowl, beat the eggs and season with salt and pepper.
3. Stir in the diced bell peppers, zucchini, onions, and shredded cheddar cheese.
4. Pour the egg mixture into the greased muffin tin, filling each cup about 3/4 full.
5. Bake for 15-20 minutes until the eggs are set and slightly golden.
6. Allow the muffins to cool for a few minutes before removing them from the tin.
7. Serve warm or refrigerate for later use.

5. Greek Yogurt and Egg Breakfast Bowl:
Ingredients:
- 2 hard-boiled eggs, sliced

- 1/2 cup Greek yoghourt
- 1/4 cup granola
- 1/4 cup mixed berries (strawberries, blueberries, raspberries)
- 1 tablespoon honey or maple syrup
- 1 tablespoon chopped nuts (almonds, walnuts, or pecans)

Instructions:
1. In a bowl, layer the Greek yoghurt at the bottom.
2. Arrange the sliced hard-boiled eggs on top of the yoghurt.
3. Sprinkle the granola and mixed berries over the eggs.
4. Drizzle with honey or maple syrup for sweetness.
5. Top with chopped nuts for added crunch.
6. Mix all the ingredients together before eating.
7. Serve chilled.

Chapter 3: Lunch Ideas for Mental Clarity

When it comes to maintaining mental clarity throughout the day, it's important to choose the right foods for lunch. Here are some comprehensive lunch ideas that can help enhance your mental clarity:

1. Salmon Salad:

Salmon is rich in omega-3 fatty acids, which are essential for brain health. To make a salmon salad, start with a bed of mixed greens and top it with grilled or baked salmon fillet. Add a variety of colourful vegetables like cherry tomatoes, cucumbers, and bell peppers. You can also include some avocado slices for healthy fats. Dress the salad with a light vinaigrette or lemon juice for added flavour.

2. Quinoa Buddha Bowl:

Quinoa is a complete protein that contains all nine essential amino acids, making it an excellent choice for brain health. To make a quinoa buddha bowl, cook quinoa according to package instructions and let it cool. In a bowl, combine cooked quinoa with a variety of roasted or steamed vegetables like broccoli, sweet potatoes, and Brussels sprouts. Add some chickpeas or grilled chicken for extra protein. Drizzle the bowl with a tahini or avocado-based dressing.

3. Mediterranean Wrap:
A Mediterranean-style lunch can provide a good balance of nutrients for mental clarity. Start with a whole wheat wrap and fill it with ingredients like grilled chicken or falafel, chopped cucumbers, tomatoes, red onions, and feta cheese. Add a dollop of hummus or tzatziki sauce for extra flavour. Wrap it up and enjoy a delicious and nutritious lunch.

4. Lentil Soup:

Lentils are packed with fibre, protein, and essential nutrients that support brain health. To make a hearty lentil soup, sauté onions, carrots, and celery in olive oil until softened. Add dried lentils, vegetable or chicken broth, and your choice of herbs and spices. Simmer until the lentils are tender. You can also add some leafy greens like spinach or kale for an extra boost of nutrients.

5. Sushi Bowl:

If you're a fan of sushi, a sushi bowl can be a convenient and nutritious lunch option. Start with a base of cooked brown rice or quinoa. Top it with sliced raw or cooked fish like salmon or tuna, along with sliced avocado, cucumber, shredded carrots, and seaweed. Drizzle with a soy sauce or a homemade sesame ginger dressing for added flavour.

Remember to stay hydrated throughout the day by drinking plenty of water or herbal tea. Avoid heavy and greasy foods that can make you feel sluggish and opt for lighter, nutrient-dense options instead. Incorporating these lunch ideas into your routine can contribute to better mental clarity and overall well-being.

Superfood Salads for Brain Power

1. Kale and Blueberry Salad:

Ingredients:

- 2 cups kale leaves, chopped
- 1 cup blueberries
- 1/4 cup walnuts, chopped
- 1/4 cup crumbled feta cheese
- 2 tablespoons lemon juice
- 1 tablespoon olive oil
- Salt and pepper to taste

Instructions:

1. In a large bowl, combine the kale, blueberries, walnuts, and feta cheese.

2. In a separate small bowl, whisk together the lemon juice, olive oil, salt, and pepper.

3. Drizzle the dressing over the salad and toss to combine.

4. Serve immediately.

2. Spinach and Quinoa Salad:

Ingredients:

- 2 cups baby spinach leaves

- 1 cup cooked quinoa

- 1/2 cup cherry tomatoes, halved

- 1/4 cup sliced almonds

- 1/4 cup crumbled goat cheese

- 2 tablespoons balsamic vinaigrette

Instructions:

1. In a large bowl, combine the spinach, quinoa, cherry tomatoes, almonds, and goat cheese.

2. Drizzle the balsamic vinaigrette over the salad and toss to combine.

3. Serve chilled.

3. Avocado and Salmon Salad:
Ingredients:
- 2 cups mixed greens
- 4 ounces grilled or baked salmon
- 1 avocado, sliced
- 1/4 cup cherry tomatoes, halved
- 2 tablespoons lemon juice
- 1 tablespoon extra virgin olive oil
- Salt and pepper to taste

Instructions:
1. Arrange the mixed greens on a plate.
2. Top with grilled or baked salmon, avocado slices, and cherry tomatoes.
3. In a small bowl, whisk together the lemon juice, olive oil, salt, and pepper.
4. Drizzle the dressing over the salad and serve.

4. Beet and Walnut Salad:
Ingredients:

- 2 cups mixed greens
- 1 medium beet, roasted and sliced
- 1/4 cup crumbled feta cheese
- 1/4 cup walnuts, chopped
- 2 tablespoons balsamic vinaigrette

Instructions:
1. Place the mixed greens in a large bowl.
2. Add the roasted beet slices, crumbled feta cheese, and chopped walnuts.
3. Drizzle the balsamic vinaigrette over the salad and toss to combine.
4. Serve chilled.

5. Quinoa and Broccoli Salad:
Ingredients:
- 2 cups cooked quinoa
- 1 cup steamed broccoli florets
- 1/4 cup dried cranberries
- 1/4 cup sunflower seeds
- 2 tablespoons lemon juice

- 1 tablespoon olive oil
- Salt and pepper to taste

Instructions:
1. In a large bowl, combine the cooked quinoa, steamed broccoli, dried cranberries, and sunflower seeds.
2. In a small bowl, whisk together the lemon juice, olive oil, salt, and pepper.
3. Drizzle the dressing over the salad and toss to combine.
4. Serve chilled.

6. Spinach and Berry Salad:
Ingredients:
- 2 cups baby spinach leaves
- 1 cup mixed berries (strawberries, blueberries, raspberries)
- 1/4 cup sliced almonds
- 1/4 cup crumbled goat cheese
- 2 tablespoons raspberry vinaigrette

Instructions:

1. Place the baby spinach leaves in a large bowl.

2. Add the mixed berries, sliced almonds, and crumbled goat cheese.

3. Drizzle the raspberry vinaigrette over the salad and toss to combine.

4. Serve chilled.

7. Quinoa and Kale Salad:

Ingredients:

- 2 cups cooked quinoa

- 2 cups kale leaves, chopped

- 1/4 cup dried cranberries

- 1/4 cup sliced almonds

- 2 tablespoons lemon juice

- 1 tablespoon extra virgin olive oil

- Salt and pepper to taste

Instructions:

1. In a large bowl, combine the cooked quinoa, chopped kale, dried cranberries, and sliced almonds.
2. In a small bowl, whisk together the lemon juice, olive oil, salt, and pepper.
3. Drizzle the dressing over the salad and toss to combine.
4. Serve chilled.

8. Sweet Potato and Chickpea Salad:
Ingredients:
- 2 cups mixed greens
- 1 medium sweet potato, roasted and cubed
- 1/2 cup cooked chickpeas
- 1/4 cup crumbled feta cheese
- 2 tablespoons lemon tahini dressing

Instructions:
1. Arrange the mixed greens on a plate.
2. Top with roasted sweet potato cubes, cooked chickpeas, and crumbled feta cheese.

3. Drizzle the lemon tahini dressing over the salad and serve.

9. Quinoa and Pomegranate Salad:
Ingredients:
- 2 cups cooked quinoa
- 1 cup pomegranate seeds
- 1/4 cup chopped pistachios
- 1/4 cup crumbled feta cheese
- 2 tablespoons lemon juice
- 1 tablespoon extra virgin olive oil
- Salt and pepper to taste

Instructions:
1. In a large bowl, combine the cooked quinoa, pomegranate seeds, chopped pistachios, and crumbled feta cheese.
2. In a small bowl, whisk together the lemon juice, olive oil, salt, and pepper.
3. Drizzle the dressing over the salad and toss to combine.

4. Serve chilled.

10. Greek Salad:

Ingredients:

- 2 cups mixed greens

- 1/2 cup cherry tomatoes, halved

- 1/4 cup sliced cucumber

- 1/4 cup Kalamata olives

- 2 tablespoons crumbled feta cheese

- 2 tablespoons Greek salad dressing

Instructions:

1. Place the mixed greens in a large bowl.

2. Add the cherry tomatoes, sliced cucumber, Kalamata olives, and crumbled feta cheese.

3. Drizzle the Greek salad dressing over the salad and toss to combine.

4. Serve chilled.

Nourishing Grain Bowls

1. Mediterranean Quinoa Bowl:

Ingredients:

- 1 cup cooked quinoa
- 1/2 cup chickpeas
- 1/4 cup diced cucumber
- 1/4 cup cherry tomatoes, halved
- 2 tablespoons sliced Kalamata olives
- 2 tablespoons crumbled feta cheese
- 1 tablespoon lemon juice
- 1 tablespoon extra virgin olive oil
- Salt and pepper to taste

Instructions:

1. In a bowl, combine the cooked quinoa, chickpeas, cucumber, cherry tomatoes, Kalamata olives, and feta cheese.

2. In a separate small bowl, whisk together the lemon juice, olive oil, salt, and pepper.

3. Drizzle the dressing over the bowl and toss to combine.

4. Serve and enjoy.

2. Teriyaki Salmon and Brown Rice Bowl:

Ingredients:

- 4 ounces grilled or baked salmon

- 1 cup cooked brown rice

- 1/2 cup steamed broccoli

- 1/4 cup shredded carrots

- 2 tablespoons teriyaki sauce

- 1 tablespoon sesame seeds

Instructions:

1. Place the cooked brown rice in a bowl.

2. Top with grilled or baked salmon, steamed broccoli, and shredded carrots.

3. Drizzle the teriyaki sauce over the bowl and sprinkle with sesame seeds.

4. Serve and enjoy.

3. Mexican Quinoa Bowl:

Ingredients:

- 1 cup cooked quinoa

- 1/2 cup black beans

- 1/4 cup diced bell peppers
- 1/4 cup diced avocado
- 2 tablespoons salsa
- 2 tablespoons chopped fresh cilantro
- 1 tablespoon lime juice
- Salt and pepper to taste

Instructions:
1. In a bowl, combine the cooked quinoa, black beans, bell peppers, avocado, salsa, and cilantro.
2. Drizzle the lime juice over the bowl and season with salt and pepper.
3. Toss to combine and serve.

4. Greek Farro Bowl:
Ingredients:
- 1 cup cooked farro
- 1/2 cup diced cucumber
- 1/4 cup cherry tomatoes, halved
- 2 tablespoons sliced Kalamata olives
- 2 tablespoons crumbled feta cheese

- 1 tablespoon lemon juice
- 1 tablespoon extra virgin olive oil
- Salt and pepper to taste

Instructions:

1. In a bowl, combine the cooked farro, cucumber, cherry tomatoes, Kalamata olives, and feta cheese.

2. In a separate small bowl, whisk together the lemon juice, olive oil, salt, and pepper.

3. Drizzle the dressing over the bowl and toss to combine.

4. Serve and enjoy.

5. Asian Quinoa Bowl:

Ingredients:

- 1 cup cooked quinoa
- 1/2 cup edamame
- 1/4 cup shredded carrots
- 1/4 cup sliced bell peppers
- 2 tablespoons soy sauce
- 1 tablespoon rice vinegar

- 1 tablespoon sesame oil
- 1 tablespoon sesame seeds

Instructions:
1. In a bowl, combine the cooked quinoa, edamame, shredded carrots, and sliced bell peppers.
2. In a separate small bowl, whisk together the soy sauce, rice vinegar, sesame oil, and sesame seeds.
3. Drizzle the dressing over the bowl and toss to combine.
4. Serve and enjoy.

6. Moroccan Couscous Bowl:
Ingredients:
- 1 cup cooked couscous
- 1/2 cup chickpeas
- 1/4 cup diced bell peppers
- 1/4 cup diced cucumber
- 2 tablespoons sliced almonds
- 1 tablespoon lemon juice
- 1 tablespoon extra virgin olive oil

- 1 teaspoon ground cumin
- Salt and pepper to taste

Instructions:

1. In a bowl, combine the cooked couscous, chickpeas, bell peppers, cucumber, and sliced almonds.

2. In a separate small bowl, whisk together the lemon juice, olive oil, ground cumin, salt, and pepper.

3. Drizzle the dressing over the bowl and toss to combine.

4. Serve and enjoy.

7. Spinach and Quinoa Bowl:

Ingredients:

- 1 cup cooked quinoa
- 1 cup baby spinach leaves
- 1/4 cup cherry tomatoes, halved
- 2 tablespoons sliced almonds
- 2 tablespoons crumbled goat cheese

- 1 tablespoon balsamic vinaigrette

Instructions:

1. In a bowl, combine the cooked quinoa, baby spinach leaves, cherry tomatoes, sliced almonds, and crumbled goat cheese.

2. Drizzle the balsamic vinaigrette over the bowl and toss to combine.

3. Serve and enjoy.

8. Thai Coconut Rice Bowl:

Ingredients:

- 1 cup cooked jasmine rice
- 1/2 cup cooked shrimp
- 1/4 cup diced bell peppers
- 1/4 cup diced pineapple
- 2 tablespoons coconut milk
- 1 tablespoon lime juice
- 1 tablespoon chopped fresh cilantro
- Salt and pepper to taste

Instructions:

1. In a bowl, combine the cooked jasmine rice, cooked shrimp, bell peppers, and pineapple.

2. In a separate small bowl, whisk together the coconut milk, lime juice, chopped cilantro, salt, and pepper.

3. Drizzle the dressing over the bowl and toss to combine.

4. Serve and enjoy.

9. Mediterranean Falafel Bowl:

Ingredients:

- 4 falafel patties
- 1 cup cooked quinoa
- 1/4 cup diced cucumber
- 1/4 cup cherry tomatoes, halved
- 2 tablespoons sliced Kalamata olives
- 2 tablespoons crumbled feta cheese
- 1 tablespoon tahini sauce

Instructions:

1. In a bowl, combine the cooked quinoa, diced cucumber, cherry tomatoes, Kalamata olives, and feta cheese.

2. Arrange the falafel patties on top of the quinoa mixture.

3. Drizzle the tahini sauce over the bowl and serve.

10. Mexican Brown Rice Bowl:

Ingredients:

- 1 cup cooked brown rice

- 1/2 cup black beans

- 1/4 cup diced bell peppers

- 1/4 cup diced avocado

- 2 tablespoons salsa

- 2 tablespoons chopped fresh cilantro

- 1 tablespoon lime juice

- Salt and pepper to taste

Instructions:

1. In a bowl, combine the cooked brown rice, black beans, bell peppers, avocado, salsa, and cilantro.

2. Drizzle the lime juice over the bowl and season with salt and pepper.

3. Toss to combine and serve.

Chapter 4: Dinner Delights for Cognitive Enhancement

1. Salmon with Lemon Dill Sauce:

Ingredients:

- 4 salmon fillets

- Juice of 1 lemon

- 2 tablespoons fresh dill, chopped

- Salt and pepper to taste

Instructions:

1. Preheat the oven to 400°F (200°C).

2. Place the salmon fillets on a baking sheet lined with parchment paper.

3. Squeeze the lemon juice over the salmon fillets and sprinkle with fresh dill, salt, and pepper.

4. Bake for 12-15 minutes or until the salmon is cooked through.

5. Serve and enjoy.

2. Spinach and Mushroom Stuffed Chicken Breast:

Ingredients:

- 4 boneless, skinless chicken breasts
- 1 cup fresh spinach leaves
- 1 cup sliced mushrooms
- 2 cloves of garlic, minced
- 1 tablespoon olive oil
- Salt and pepper to taste

Instructions:

1. Preheat the oven to 375°F (190°C).

2. In a skillet, heat the olive oil over medium heat.

3. Add the minced garlic and sauté for 1-2 minutes until fragrant.

4. Add the sliced mushrooms and cook until they release their moisture and become tender.

5. Add the fresh spinach leaves and cook until wilted.

6. Slice a pocket into each chicken breast and stuff with the spinach and mushroom mixture.

7. Season the chicken breasts with salt and pepper.

8. Place the stuffed chicken breasts on a baking sheet and bake for 25-30 minutes or until cooked through.

9. Serve and enjoy.

3. Quinoa Stuffed Bell Peppers:

Ingredients:

- 4 bell peppers (any colour)

- 1 cup cooked quinoa

- 1/2 cup black beans

- 1/2 cup corn kernels

- 1/4 cup diced tomatoes

- 1/4 cup shredded cheddar cheese

- 1 tablespoon olive oil

- 1 teaspoon cumin

- Salt and pepper to taste

Instructions:

1. Preheat the oven to 375°F (190°C).

2. Cut the tops off the bell peppers and remove the seeds and membranes.

3. In a bowl, mix together the cooked quinoa, black beans, corn kernels, diced tomatoes, olive oil, cumin, salt, and pepper.
4. Stuff the bell peppers with the quinoa mixture and place them in a baking dish.
5. Sprinkle the shredded cheddar cheese over the stuffed bell peppers.
6. Bake for 25-30 minutes or until the peppers are tender and the cheese is melted and golden.
7. Serve and enjoy.

4. Lentil and Vegetable Curry:
Ingredients:
- 1 cup lentils, cooked
- 1 cup mixed vegetables (carrots, peas, bell peppers, etc.)
- 1 onion, chopped
- 2 cloves of garlic, minced
- 1 tablespoon curry powder
- 1 tablespoon tomato paste
- 1 can (14 oz) coconut milk

- 1 tablespoon olive oil
- Salt and pepper to taste

Instructions:

1. In a large skillet, heat the olive oil over medium heat.

2. Add the chopped onion and minced garlic and sauté until the onion is translucent.

3. Add the curry powder and tomato paste and cook for 1-2 minutes.

4. Add the mixed vegetables and cook until they are tender.

5. Stir in the cooked lentils and coconut milk.

6. Simmer for 10-15 minutes to allow the flavours to meld.

7. Season with salt and pepper to taste.

8. Serve the lentil and vegetable curry over cooked rice or with naan bread.

9. Enjoy.

5. Baked Cod with Garlic Butter:

Ingredients:
- 4 cod fillets
- 4 tablespoons unsalted butter, melted
- 2 cloves of garlic, minced
- Juice of 1 lemon
- Salt and pepper to taste

Instructions:
1. Preheat the oven to 400°F (200°C).
2. Place the cod fillets on a baking sheet lined with parchment paper.
3. In a small bowl, mix together the melted butter, minced garlic, lemon juice, salt, and pepper.
4. Drizzle the garlic butter mixture over the cod fillets.
5. Bake for 12-15 minutes or until the cod is opaque and flakes easily with a fork.
6. Serve and enjoy.

6. Grilled Chicken and Vegetable Skewers:
Ingredients:

- 4 boneless, skinless chicken breasts, cut into cubes
- 1 zucchini, sliced
- 1 bell pepper, cut into chunks
- 1 red onion, cut into chunks
- 2 tablespoons olive oil
- 2 teaspoons Italian seasoning
- Salt and pepper to taste

Instructions:
1. Preheat the grill to medium-high heat.
2. Thread the chicken, zucchini, bell pepper, and red onion onto skewers.
3. In a small bowl, whisk together the olive oil, Italian seasoning, salt, and pepper.
4. Brush the skewers with the olive oil mixture.
5. Grill the skewers for 10-12 minutes, turning occasionally, until the chicken is cooked through.
6. Serve and enjoy.

7. Sweet Potato and Chickpea Curry:
Ingredients:

- 2 sweet potatoes, peeled and cubed
- 1 can (14 oz) chickpeas, drained and rinsed
- 1 onion, chopped
- 2 cloves of garlic, minced
- 1 tablespoon curry powder
- 1 can (14 oz) coconut milk
- 1 tablespoon olive oil
- Salt and pepper to taste

Instructions:

1. In a large skillet, heat the olive oil over medium heat.

2. Add the chopped onion and minced garlic and sauté until the onion is translucent.

3. Add the curry powder and cook for 1-2 minutes.

4. Add the cubed sweet potatoes and cook until they start to soften.

5. Stir in the chickpeas and coconut milk.

6. Simmer for 15-20 minutes or until the sweet potatoes are tender.

7. Season with salt and pepper to taste.

8. Serve the sweet potato and chickpea curry over cooked rice or with naan bread.

9. Enjoy.

8. Beef Stir-Fry with Broccoli:

Ingredients:

- 1 pound beef sirloin, thinly sliced
- 2 cups broccoli florets
- 1 bell pepper, sliced
- 1 onion, sliced
- 2 cloves of garlic, minced
- 2 tablespoons soy sauce
- 1 tablespoon oyster sauce
- 1 tablespoon cornstarch
- 2 tablespoons vegetable oil
- Salt and pepper to taste

Instructions:

1. In a small bowl, whisk together the soy sauce, oyster sauce, cornstarch, salt, and pepper.

2. In a large skillet or wok, heat the vegetable oil over high heat.
3. Add the minced garlic and stir-fry for 1 minute.
4. Add the beef slices and stir-fry until browned.
5. Add the broccoli florets, bell pepper, and onion.
6. Stir-fry for 3-4 minutes or until the vegetables are crisp-tender.
7. Pour the sauce mixture over the stir-fry and cook for an additional 2 minutes, until the sauce thickens.
8. Serve over cooked rice or noodles.
9. Enjoy.

9. Shrimp and Vegetable Stir-Fry:
Ingredients:
- 1 pound shrimp, peeled and deveined
- 2 cups mixed vegetables (carrots, bell peppers, snap peas, etc.)
- 1 onion, sliced
- 2 cloves of garlic, minced
- 2 tablespoons soy sauce

- 1 tablespoon hoisin sauce

- 1 tablespoon cornstarch

- 2 tablespoons vegetable oil

- Salt and pepper to taste

Instructions:

1. In a small bowl, whisk together the soy sauce, hoisin sauce, cornstarch, salt, and pepper.

2. In a large skillet or wok, heat the vegetable oil over high heat.

3. Add the minced garlic and stir-fry for 1 minute.

4. Add the shrimp and stir-fry until pink and cooked through.

5. Add the mixed vegetables and onion.

6. Stir-fry for 3-4 minutes or until the vegetables are crisp-tender.

7. Pour the sauce mixture over the stir-fry and cook for an additional 2 minutes, until the sauce thickens.

8. Serve over cooked rice or noodles.

9. Enjoy.

10. Veggie Packed Pasta Primavera:

Ingredients:

- 8 ounces whole wheat pasta

- 2 cups mixed vegetables (broccoli, zucchini, bell peppers, etc.)

- 1 onion, sliced

- 2 cloves of garlic, minced

- 2 tablespoons olive oil

- 1/4 cup grated Parmesan cheese

- Salt and pepper to taste

Instructions:

1. Cook the pasta according to package instructions until al dente. Drain and set aside.

2. In a large skillet, heat the olive oil over medium heat.

3. Add the sliced onion and minced garlic and sauté until the onion is translucent.

4. Add the mixed vegetables and cook until they are tender-crisp.

5. Season with salt and pepper to taste.

6. Add the cooked pasta to the skillet and toss to combine.

7. Sprinkle with grated Parmesan cheese and stir to melt the cheese.

8. Serve and enjoy.

Plant-Based Meals Bursting with Brain-Boosting Ingredients

1. Blueberry Spinach Smoothie Bowl:

   Ingredients:

   - 1 cup spinach

   - 1 cup frozen blueberries

   - 1 ripe banana

   - 1 tablespoon chia seeds

   - 1 cup almond milk

   Instructions:

   1. Blend all the ingredients until smooth.

2. Pour the mixture into a bowl and top with your favourite toppings like granola, nuts, and more blueberries.

2. Quinoa Salad with Avocado and Walnuts:
   Ingredients:
   - 1 cup cooked quinoa
   - 1 avocado, diced
   - 1/4 cup walnuts, chopped
   - 1/4 cup dried cranberries
   - 2 tablespoons lemon juice
   - 1 tablespoon olive oil
   - Salt and pepper to taste

   Instructions:
1. In a bowl, combine the cooked quinoa, avocado, walnuts, and dried cranberries.
2. In a separate small bowl, whisk together the lemon juice, olive oil, salt, and pepper.
3. Drizzle the dressing over the quinoa mixture and toss to combine.

3. Lentil and Vegetable Stir-Fry:
   Ingredients:
   - 1 cup cooked lentils
   - 1 cup mixed vegetables (broccoli, bell peppers, carrots, etc.)
   - 2 cloves garlic, minced
   - 1 tablespoon soy sauce
   - 1 tablespoon sesame oil
   - 1 tablespoon maple syrup

   Instructions:
1. Heat the sesame oil in a pan over medium heat.
2. Add the minced garlic and sauté for 1-2 minutes.
3. Add the mixed vegetables and cook until tender.
4. Stir in the cooked lentils, soy sauce, and maple syrup. Cook for an additional 2-3 minutes.

4. Sweet Potato and Chickpea Curry:
   Ingredients:
   - 2 sweet potatoes, peeled and cubed

- 1 can chickpeas, drained and rinsed
- 1 onion, diced
- 2 cloves garlic, minced
- 1 tablespoon curry powder
- 1 can coconut milk
- Salt and pepper to taste

Instructions:

1. In a large pot, sauté the onion and garlic until fragrant.

2. Add the sweet potatoes, chickpeas, curry powder, coconut milk, salt, and pepper.

3. Bring to a boil, then reduce heat and simmer until the sweet potatoes are tender.

5. Spinach and Mushroom Omelette:
Ingredients:
- 1 cup spinach, chopped
- 1/2 cup mushrooms, sliced
- 4-5 cherry tomatoes, halved

- 3-4 vegan eggs (made from chickpea flour or tofu)

- Salt and pepper to taste

Instructions:

1. In a non-stick pan, sauté the mushrooms until they release their moisture.

2. Add the spinach and cherry tomatoes to the pan and cook until wilted.

3. In a separate bowl, whisk the vegan eggs with salt and pepper.

4. Pour the egg mixture over the vegetables in the pan and cook until set.

6. Chia Seed Pudding with Berries:

Ingredients:

- 2 tablespoons chia seeds

- 1 cup almond milk

- 1 tablespoon maple syrup

- Fresh berries for topping

Instructions:

1. In a jar or bowl, mix together the chia seeds, almond milk, and maple syrup.

2. Stir well and refrigerate overnight or for at least 2 hours.

3. Serve with fresh berries on top.

7. Quinoa Stuffed Bell Peppers:

Ingredients:

- 4 bell peppers
- 1 cup cooked quinoa
- 1 cup black beans, drained and rinsed
- 1/2 cup corn kernels
- 1/2 cup diced tomatoes
- 1/4 cup chopped fresh cilantro
- 1 teaspoon cumin
- Salt and pepper to taste

Instructions:

1. Preheat the oven to 375°F (190°C).

2. Cut off the tops of the bell peppers and remove the seeds.

3. In a bowl, mix together the cooked quinoa, black beans, corn, tomatoes, cilantro, cumin, salt, and pepper.

4. Stuff the mixture into the bell peppers and place them in a baking dish.

5. Bake for 25-30 minutes or until the bell peppers are tender.

8. Broccoli and Almond Stir-Fry:

Ingredients:

- 2 cups broccoli florets
- 1/4 cup sliced almonds
- 2 cloves garlic, minced
- 2 tablespoons soy sauce
- 1 tablespoon sesame oil
- 1 tablespoon maple syrup

Instructions:

1. Heat the sesame oil in a pan over medium heat.

2. Add the minced garlic and sauté for 1-2 minutes.

3. Add the broccoli florets and cook until tender.

4. Stir in the sliced almonds, soy sauce, and maple syrup. Cook for an additional 2-3 minutes.

9. Kale and Quinoa Salad with Lemon Tahini Dressing:

Ingredients:

- 2 cups kale, chopped
- 1 cup cooked quinoa
- 1/4 cup sliced almonds
- 1/4 cup dried cranberries
- 2 tablespoons lemon juice
- 2 tablespoons tahini
- 1 tablespoon maple syrup
- Salt and pepper to taste

Instructions:

1. In a large bowl, combine the chopped kale, cooked quinoa, sliced almonds, and dried cranberries.

2. In a small bowl, whisk together the lemon juice, tahini, maple syrup, salt, and pepper.

3. Drizzle the dressing over the salad and toss to combine.

10. Vegan Lentil Bolognese:

Ingredients:

- 1 cup dried lentils

- 1 onion, diced

- 2 cloves garlic, minced

- 1 carrot, grated

- 1 can diced tomatoes

- 1 tablespoon tomato paste

- 1 tablespoon Italian seasoning

- Salt and pepper to taste

- Whole wheat or gluten-free pasta, cooked, for serving

Instructions:

1. Cook the lentils according to package instructions and set aside.

2. In a large pan, sauté the onion and garlic until fragrant.

3. Add the grated carrot and cook until softened.

4. Stir in the diced tomatoes, tomato paste, Italian seasoning, salt, and pepper.

5. Add the cooked lentils and simmer for 10-15 minutes.

6. Serve the lentil Bolognese over cooked pasta.

Wholesome Meat and Poultry Recipes for Mental Wellness

1. Grilled Salmon with Lemon and Dill:

Ingredients:

- 4 salmon fillets

- 2 lemons, sliced

- Fresh dill

- Salt and pepper to taste

Instructions:

1. Preheat the grill to medium heat.

2. Season the salmon fillets with salt and pepper.

3. Place the salmon on the grill and top each fillet with a slice of lemon and fresh dill.

4. Grill for about 5-6 minutes per side or until the salmon is cooked through.

2. Baked Chicken Breast with Herbs:
Ingredients:
- 4 boneless, skinless chicken breasts
- 2 tablespoons olive oil
- 1 teaspoon dried thyme
- 1 teaspoon dried rosemary
- Salt and pepper to taste

Instructions:
1. Preheat the oven to 400°F (200°C).

2. Rub the chicken breasts with olive oil, dried thyme, dried rosemary, salt, and pepper.

3. Place the chicken breasts on a baking sheet and bake for 20-25 minutes or until cooked through.

3. Turkey and Vegetable Stir-Fry:

Ingredients:

- 1 pound ground turkey
- 2 cups mixed vegetables (broccoli, bell peppers, carrots, etc.)
- 2 cloves garlic, minced
- 2 tablespoons soy sauce
- 1 tablespoon sesame oil
- 1 tablespoon maple syrup

Instructions:

1. Heat the sesame oil in a pan over medium heat.

2. Add the minced garlic and sauté for 1-2 minutes.

3. Add the ground turkey and cook until browned.

4. Stir in the mixed vegetables, soy sauce, and maple syrup. Cook for an additional 5-7 minutes.

4. Herb-Roasted Chicken Thighs:

Ingredients:

- 4 chicken thighs, bone-in and skin-on

- 2 tablespoons olive oil
- 1 teaspoon dried thyme
- 1 teaspoon dried rosemary
- Salt and pepper to taste

Instructions:

1. Preheat the oven to 425°F (220°C).

2. Rub the chicken thighs with olive oil, dried thyme, dried rosemary, salt, and pepper.

3. Place the chicken thighs on a baking sheet, skin-side up, and roast for 30-35 minutes or until golden and cooked through.

5. Lemon Garlic Shrimp Stir-Fry:

Ingredients:
- 1 pound shrimp, peeled and deveined
- 2 cups mixed vegetables (broccoli, bell peppers, carrots, etc.)
- 2 cloves garlic, minced
- 2 tablespoons lemon juice
- 1 tablespoon olive oil

- Salt and pepper to taste

Instructions:

1. Heat the olive oil in a pan over medium heat.

2. Add the minced garlic and sauté for 1-2 minutes.

3. Add the shrimp and cook until pink and opaque.

4. Stir in the mixed vegetables, lemon juice, salt, and pepper. Cook for an additional 3-4 minutes.

6. Herb-Marinated Grilled Chicken Skewers:
Ingredients:
- 1 pound chicken breast, cut into cubes
- 2 tablespoons olive oil
- 1 teaspoon dried oregano
- 1 teaspoon dried basil
- Salt and pepper to taste

Instructions:

1. In a bowl, combine the olive oil, dried oregano, dried basil, salt, and pepper.

2. Add the chicken cubes to the bowl and toss to coat.

3. Thread the chicken onto skewers and grill for about 10-12 minutes, turning occasionally, until cooked through.

7. Beef and Broccoli Stir-Fry:

Ingredients:

- 1 pound beef sirloin, thinly sliced
- 2 cups broccoli florets
- 2 cloves garlic, minced
- 2 tablespoons soy sauce
- 1 tablespoon sesame oil
- 1 tablespoon maple syrup

Instructions:

1. Heat the sesame oil in a pan over medium heat.

2. Add the minced garlic and sauté for 1-2 minutes.

3. Add the beef sirloin and cook until browned.

4. Stir in the broccoli florets, soy sauce, and maple syrup. Cook for an additional 5-7 minutes.

8. Lemon Herb Roasted Turkey Breast:
Ingredients:
- 1 turkey breast, bone-in and skin-on
- 2 tablespoons olive oil
- 2 tablespoons lemon juice
- 1 teaspoon dried thyme
- 1 teaspoon dried rosemary
- Salt and pepper to taste

Instructions:
1. Preheat the oven to 350°F (175°C).

2. In a small bowl, whisk together the olive oil, lemon juice, dried thyme, dried rosemary, salt, and pepper.

3. Rub the turkey breast with the mixture and place it in a roasting pan.

4. Roast for about 2-2.5 hours or until the internal temperature reaches 165°F (75°C).

9. Teriyaki Glazed Salmon:
Ingredients:
- 4 salmon fillets
- 1/4 cup soy sauce
- 2 tablespoons maple syrup
- 1 tablespoon rice vinegar
- 1 teaspoon minced ginger
- 1 clove garlic, minced

Instructions:
1. Preheat the oven to 400°F (200°C).

2. In a small saucepan, combine the soy sauce, maple syrup, rice vinegar, minced ginger, and minced garlic.

3. Cook over medium heat until the mixture thickens slightly.

4. Place the salmon fillets on a baking sheet and brush them with the teriyaki glaze.

5. Bake for 12-15 minutes or until the salmon is cooked through.

10. Herb-Marinated Grilled Steak:
Ingredients:
- 1 pound steak (such as sirloin or ribeye)
- 2 tablespoons olive oil
- 1 teaspoon dried thyme
- 1 teaspoon dried rosemary
- Salt and pepper to taste

Instructions:
1. In a bowl, combine the olive oil, dried thyme, dried rosemary, salt, and pepper.
2. Place the steak in a shallow dish and pour the marinade over it. Let it marinate for at least 30 minutes.
3. Preheat the grill to medium-high heat.
4. Grill the steak for about 4-5 minutes per side for medium-rare or until desired doneness.

Chapter 5: Snacks and Appetisers to Stimulate Brain Function

1. Blueberry Yogurt Parfait:

Ingredients:

- 1 cup Greek yoghourt

- 1/2 cup fresh blueberries

- 2 tablespoons granola

- 1 tablespoon honey

Instructions:

1. In a glass or bowl, layer Greek yoghurt, blueberries, and granola.

2. Drizzle with honey and enjoy.

2. Avocado Toast:

Ingredients:

- 2 slices whole grain bread

- 1 ripe avocado

- 1 tablespoon lemon juice

- Salt and pepper to taste

Instructions:

1. Toast the bread slices until golden brown.

2. In a bowl, mash the avocado with lemon juice, salt, and pepper.

3. Spread the mashed avocado onto the toasted bread slices.

4. Optional: Top with additional toppings like cherry tomatoes, feta cheese, or smoked salmon.

3. Spinach and Feta Stuffed Mushrooms:

Ingredients:

- 10 large mushrooms

- 1 cup fresh spinach, chopped

- 1/2 cup feta cheese, crumbled

- 1 clove garlic, minced

- 1 tablespoon olive oil

- Salt and pepper to taste

Instructions:

1. Preheat the oven to 375°F (190°C).

2. Remove the stems from the mushrooms and set them aside.

3. In a pan, heat olive oil over medium heat.

4. Add minced garlic and chopped mushroom stems. Cook for 3-4 minutes.

5. Add chopped spinach and cook until wilted.

6. Remove from heat and stir in feta cheese, salt, and pepper.

7. Stuff the mushroom caps with the spinach and feta mixture.

8. Place the stuffed mushrooms on a baking sheet and bake for 15-20 minutes or until the mushrooms are tender.

4. Trail Mix:

Ingredients:

- 1 cup mixed nuts (almonds, walnuts, cashews)

- 1/2 cup dried fruits (raisins, cranberries, apricots)

- 1/4 cup dark chocolate chips

Instructions:

1. In a bowl, combine mixed nuts, dried fruits, and dark chocolate chips.

2. Mix well and portion into individual servings for a quick and brain-boosting snack.

5. Guacamole with Veggie Sticks:

Ingredients:

- 2 ripe avocados

- 1 small tomato, diced

- 1/4 cup red onion, finely chopped

- 1 clove garlic, minced

- Juice of 1 lime

- Salt and pepper to taste

- Assorted veggie sticks (carrots, cucumber, bell peppers) for dipping

Instructions:

1. In a bowl, mash the avocados with a fork.

2. Add diced tomato, red onion, minced garlic, lime juice, salt, and pepper. Mix well.

3. Serve the guacamole with veggie sticks for a brain-boosting and nutritious snack.

6. Smoked Salmon Roll-Ups:

Ingredients:

- 4 slices smoked salmon

- 1/4 cup cream cheese

- 2 tablespoons capers

- Fresh dill for garnish

Instructions:

1. Lay the smoked salmon slices flat on a cutting board.

2. Spread a thin layer of cream cheese onto each slice.

3. Sprinkle capers evenly over the cream cheese.

4. Roll up the salmon slices and secure with toothpicks.

5. Garnish with fresh dill and serve.

7. Hummus with Whole Grain Crackers:
   Ingredients:
   - 1 cup canned chickpeas, drained and rinsed
   - 2 tablespoons tahini
   - 2 tablespoons lemon juice
   - 1 clove garlic
   - 2 tablespoons olive oil
   - Salt and pepper to taste
   - Whole grain crackers for dipping

   Instructions:
   1. In a food processor, combine chickpeas, tahini, lemon juice, garlic, olive oil, salt, and pepper.
   2. Process until smooth and creamy.
   3. Serve the hummus with whole grain crackers for a brain-boosting snack.

8. Veggie Sushi Rolls:
   Ingredients:
   - 4 sheets of nori (seaweed)

- 2 cups cooked sushi rice

- Assorted veggies (carrots, cucumber, avocado, bell peppers), julienned

- Soy sauce and wasabi for dipping

Instructions:

1. Place a sheet of nori on a bamboo sushi mat or a clean kitchen towel.

2. Spread a thin layer of sushi rice evenly over the nori, leaving a small border at the top.

3. Arrange julienned veggies in a line across the rice.

4. Roll the sushi tightly, using the sushi mat or towel to help. Moisten the border with water to seal.

5. Slice the sushi roll into bite-sized pieces.

6. Serve with soy sauce and wasabi for dipping.

9. Berry Spinach Smoothie:

Ingredients:

- 1 cup fresh spinach

- 1/2 cup mixed berries (strawberries, blueberries, raspberries)
- 1/2 banana
- 1 cup almond milk (or any preferred milk)
- 1 tablespoon chia seeds (optional)

Instructions:

1. Place all ingredients in a blender and blend until smooth and creamy.

2. Pour into a glass and enjoy the brain-boosting goodness.

10. Dark Chocolate Energy Balls:

Ingredients:
- 1 cup pitted dates
- 1/2 cup almonds
- 2 tablespoons unsweetened cocoa powder
- 1 tablespoon honey
- 1/4 cup shredded coconut (for coating)

Instructions:

1. In a food processor, combine dates, almonds, cocoa powder, and honey.

2. Process until the mixture comes together and forms a sticky dough.

3. Roll the dough into small balls and coat them with shredded coconut.

4. Place the energy balls in the refrigerator for at least 30 minutes before serving.

Veggie-Based Dips and Spreads

1. Roasted Red Pepper Hummus:

Ingredients:

- 1 can chickpeas, drained and rinsed

- 1 roasted red pepper, peeled and seeded

- 2 tablespoons tahini

- 2 tablespoons lemon juice

- 1 clove garlic

- 2 tablespoons olive oil

- Salt and pepper to taste

Instructions:

1. In a food processor, combine chickpeas, roasted red pepper, tahini, lemon juice, garlic, olive oil, salt, and pepper.

2. Process until smooth and creamy.

3. Serve as a dip with pita chips or veggies.

2. Spinach and Artichoke Dip:

Ingredients:

- 1 cup frozen spinach, thawed and squeezed dry
- 1 cup canned artichoke hearts, chopped
- 1 cup cream cheese
- 1/2 cup sour cream
- 1/2 cup grated Parmesan cheese
- 1/2 cup shredded mozzarella cheese
- 1 clove garlic, minced
- Salt and pepper to taste

Instructions:

1. Preheat the oven to 375°F (190°C).

2. In a bowl, mix together spinach, artichoke hearts, cream cheese, sour cream, Parmesan cheese, mozzarella cheese, garlic, salt, and pepper.

3. Transfer the mixture to a baking dish and bake for 20-25 minutes or until bubbly and golden.

4. Serve with tortilla chips or bread slices.

3. Baba Ganoush:

Ingredients:

- 2 large eggplants
- 1/4 cup tahini
- 2 tablespoons lemon juice
- 1 clove garlic, minced
- 2 tablespoons olive oil
- Salt and pepper to taste

Instructions:

1. Preheat the oven to 400°F (200°C).

2. Pierce the eggplants with a fork and place them on a baking sheet.

3. Roast the eggplants in the oven for 45-50 minutes or until the skins are charred and the flesh is soft.

4. Let the eggplants cool, then peel off the skin and discard.

5. In a food processor, blend the roasted eggplant flesh, tahini, lemon juice, garlic, olive oil, salt, and pepper until smooth.

6. Serve as a dip with pita bread or veggies.

4. Cucumber Yogurt Dip:
Ingredients:
- 1 cup Greek yoghourt
- 1 small cucumber, grated and squeezed dry
- 1 clove garlic, minced
- 1 tablespoon lemon juice
- 1 tablespoon chopped fresh dill
- Salt and pepper to taste

Instructions:

1. In a bowl, mix together Greek yoghurt, grated cucumber, minced garlic, lemon juice, chopped dill, salt, and pepper.

2. Refrigerate for at least 1 hour before serving.

3. Serve with pita chips or veggie sticks.

5. Roasted Beet and Goat Cheese Spread:

Ingredients:

- 2 medium beets, roasted and peeled

- 4 ounces goat cheese

- 2 tablespoons chopped fresh herbs (such as dill, parsley, or chives)

- Salt and pepper to taste

Instructions:

1. In a food processor, blend roasted beets, goat cheese, chopped herbs, salt, and pepper until smooth and well combined.

2. Transfer the spread to a serving bowl.

3. Serve with crackers or bread slices.

6. Zucchini and Feta Dip:

Ingredients:

- 2 medium zucchinis, grated and squeezed dry

- 1/2 cup crumbled feta cheese

- 1/4 cup Greek yoghourt

- 1 clove garlic, minced

- 1 tablespoon lemon juice

- 1 tablespoon chopped fresh mint

- Salt and pepper to taste

Instructions:

1. In a bowl, combine grated zucchini, feta cheese, Greek yoghourt, minced garlic, lemon juice, chopped mint, salt, and pepper.

2. Mix well until all ingredients are evenly incorporated.

3. Refrigerate for at least 30 minutes before serving.

4. Serve with pita bread or veggie sticks.

7. Carrot and Ginger Spread:

Ingredients:
- 2 large carrots, grated
- 1 tablespoon grated fresh ginger
- 1/4 cup cream cheese
- 2 tablespoons Greek yoghourt
- 1 tablespoon lemon juice
- Salt and pepper to taste

Instructions:
1. In a bowl, mix together grated carrots, grated ginger, cream cheese, Greek yoghurt, lemon juice, salt, and pepper.
2. Stir until well combined.
3. Refrigerate for at least 1 hour before serving.
4. Serve with crackers or bread slices.

8. Spicy Roasted Tomato Salsa:
Ingredients:
- 4 medium tomatoes, halved
- 1 small onion, quartered
- 2 cloves garlic

- 1 jalapeno pepper, seeded and chopped
- 2 tablespoons lime juice
- 1/4 cup chopped fresh cilantro
- Salt and pepper to taste

Instructions:

1. Preheat the oven to 400°F (200°C).

2. Place the tomato halves, onion quarters, and garlic cloves on a baking sheet.

3. Roast in the oven for 20-25 minutes or until the tomatoes are soft and slightly charred.

4. Let the roasted vegetables cool, then transfer them to a food processor.

5. Add chopped jalapeno, lime juice, chopped cilantro, salt, and pepper to the food processor.

6. Pulse until the salsa reaches your desired consistency.

7. Serve with tortilla chips or use as a topping for tacos.

9. Edamame and Mint Dip:

Ingredients:
- 1 cup shelled edamame, cooked and cooled
- 1/4 cup fresh mint leaves
- 2 tablespoons Greek yoghourt
- 1 tablespoon lemon juice
- 1 clove garlic, minced
- 1 tablespoon olive oil
- Salt and pepper to taste

Instructions:
1. In a food processor, blend cooked edamame, mint leaves, Greek yoghourt, lemon juice, minced garlic, olive oil, salt, and pepper until smooth.
2. Transfer the dip to a serving bowl.
3. Serve with pita chips or veggie sticks.

10. Sweet Potato and Black Bean Dip:
Ingredients:
- 1 large sweet potato, roasted and peeled
- 1 can black beans, drained and rinsed
- 1/4 cup Greek yoghourt

- 1 tablespoon lime juice

- 1 teaspoon ground cumin

- 1/2 teaspoon chilli powder

- Salt and pepper to taste

Instructions:

1. In a food processor, blend roasted sweet potato, black beans, Greek yoghurt, lime juice, ground cumin, chilli powder, salt, and pepper until smooth and well combined.

2. Transfer the dip to a serving bowl.

3. Serve with tortilla chips or veggie sticks.

Brain-Enhancing Bites and Finger Foods

1. Blueberry and Walnut Energy Balls:

Ingredients:

- 1 cup rolled oats

- 1/2 cup almond butter

- 1/4 cup honey

- 1/4 cup dried blueberries

- 1/4 cup chopped walnuts

- 1 tablespoon ground flaxseed

Instructions:

1. In a mixing bowl, combine rolled oats, almond butter, honey, dried blueberries, chopped walnuts, and ground flaxseed.

2. Mix well until all ingredients are evenly incorporated.

3. Roll the mixture into bite-sized balls.

4. Refrigerate for at least 1 hour before serving.

2. Smoked Salmon and Avocado Roll-ups:

Ingredients:

- 4 slices smoked salmon

- 1 ripe avocado, sliced

- 2 tablespoons cream cheese

- 1 tablespoon lemon juice

- Salt and pepper to taste

Instructions:

1. Lay a slice of smoked salmon on a clean surface.

2. Spread a thin layer of cream cheese on the salmon slice.

3. Place a few slices of avocado on top of the cream cheese.

4. Drizzle with lemon juice and season with salt and pepper.

5. Roll up the salmon slice tightly.

6. Repeat with the remaining ingredients.

7. Slice each roll-up into bite-sized pieces.

8. Serve chilled.

3. Kale Chips:

Ingredients:

- 1 bunch kale, stems removed and leaves torn into bite-sized pieces

- 2 tablespoons olive oil

- Salt and pepper to taste

Instructions:

1. Preheat the oven to 350°F (175°C).

2. In a large bowl, toss kale leaves with olive oil, salt, and pepper.

3. Spread the kale leaves in a single layer on a baking sheet.

4. Bake for 10-15 minutes or until the kale chips are crispy.

5. Let them cool before serving.

4. Quinoa Stuffed Bell Peppers:

Ingredients:

- 4 bell peppers, tops removed and seeds removed
- 1 cup cooked quinoa
- 1 cup cooked black beans
- 1/2 cup diced tomatoes
- 1/2 cup chopped spinach
- 1/4 cup shredded cheddar cheese
- 1 teaspoon cumin
- Salt and pepper to taste

Instructions:

1. Preheat the oven to 375°F (190°C).

2. In a mixing bowl, combine cooked quinoa, black beans, diced tomatoes, chopped spinach, shredded cheddar cheese, cumin, salt, and pepper.

3. Stuff each bell pepper with the quinoa mixture.

4. Place the stuffed bell peppers in a baking dish.

5. Bake for 25-30 minutes or until the peppers are tender and the filling is heated through.

6. Let them cool slightly before serving.

5. Trail Mix:

Ingredients:

- 1 cup mixed nuts (such as almonds, walnuts, and cashews)

- 1/2 cup dried fruits (such as cranberries, raisins, and apricots)

- 1/2 cup dark chocolate chips

- 1/4 cup pumpkin seeds

- 1/4 cup unsweetened coconut flakes

Instructions:

1. In a bowl, mix together mixed nuts, dried fruits, dark chocolate chips, pumpkin seeds, and coconut flakes.

2. Toss until all ingredients are well combined.

3. Store in an airtight container for snacking on the go.

6. Greek Yoghourt Parfait:

Ingredients:

- 1 cup Greek yoghourt

- 1/2 cup mixed berries (such as blueberries, raspberries, and strawberries)

- 1/4 cup granola

- 1 tablespoon honey

Instructions:

1. In a glass or jar, layer Greek yoghourt, mixed berries, granola, and drizzle with honey.

2. Repeat the layers until all ingredients are used.

3. Serve chilled.

7. Spinach and Feta Stuffed Mushrooms:
  Ingredients:
   - 12 large mushrooms, stems removed and caps cleaned
   - 2 cups chopped spinach
   - 1/2 cup crumbled feta cheese
   - 2 cloves garlic, minced
   - 2 tablespoons olive oil
   - Salt and pepper to taste

Instructions:
1. Preheat the oven to 375°F (190°C).
2. In a skillet, heat olive oil over medium heat.
3. Add minced garlic and chopped spinach to the skillet.
4. Sauté until the spinach is wilted.
5. Remove from heat and stir in crumbled feta cheese, salt, and pepper.
6. Stuff each mushroom cap with the spinach and feta mixture.
7. Place the stuffed mushrooms on a baking sheet.

8. Bake for 15-20 minutes or until the mushrooms are tender.

9. Let them cool slightly before serving.

8. Chia Pudding Cups:

Ingredients:

- 1/4 cup chia seeds

- 1 cup almond milk

- 1 tablespoon honey

- 1/2 teaspoon vanilla extract

- Fresh fruits for topping (such as berries or sliced bananas)

Instructions:

1. In a bowl, mix together chia seeds, almond milk, honey, and vanilla extract.

2. Stir well to combine and let the mixture sit for 10 minutes.

3. Stir again to break up any clumps of chia seeds.

4. Divide the chia pudding into small cups or jars.

5. Refrigerate for at least 2 hours or overnight.

6. Top with fresh fruits before serving.

9. Spinach and Cheese Quesadillas:
Ingredients:
- 4 large whole wheat tortillas
- 2 cups fresh spinach leaves
- 1 cup shredded mozzarella cheese
- 1/2 cup diced tomatoes
- 1/4 cup chopped red onion
- Salt and pepper to taste

Instructions:
1. Place one tortilla on a clean surface.

2. Layer spinach leaves, shredded mozzarella cheese, diced tomatoes, chopped red onion, salt, and pepper on top of the tortilla.

3. Cover with another tortilla.

4. Heat a skillet over medium heat and cook the quesadilla for 2-3 minutes on each side or until the cheese is melted and the tortilla is crispy.

5. Repeat with the remaining ingredients.

6. Let them cool slightly before slicing into wedges.

7. Serve warm.

10. Dark Chocolate Covered Almonds:

Ingredients:

- 1 cup whole almonds

- 4 ounces dark chocolate, chopped

- 1/2 teaspoon coconut oil

Instructions:

1. In a microwave-safe bowl, melt the dark chocolate and coconut oil together in 30-second intervals, stirring in between, until smooth.

2. Dip each almond into the melted chocolate, coating it completely.

3. Place the chocolate-covered almonds on a parchment-lined baking sheet.

4. Let them cool and harden at room temperature.

5. Store in an airtight container for snacking.

Chapter 6: Desserts and Treats for Cognitive Indulgence

1. Dark Chocolate Bark with Almonds and Blueberries:

Ingredients:

- 8 ounces dark chocolate, chopped

- 1/2 cup almonds, chopped

- 1/2 cup dried blueberries

Instructions:

1. Melt the dark chocolate in a microwave-safe bowl or using a double boiler.

2. Stir in the chopped almonds and dried blueberries.

3. Pour the mixture onto a parchment-lined baking sheet and spread it evenly.

4. Allow it to cool and harden in the refrigerator for about 1 hour.

5. Once hardened, break the bark into smaller pieces and enjoy.

2. Matcha Green Tea Chia Pudding:
Ingredients:
- 2 tablespoons chia seeds
- 1 cup almond milk (or any other milk of your choice)
- 1 teaspoon matcha green tea powder
- 1 tablespoon honey or maple syrup (optional)

Instructions:
1. In a bowl, whisk together the chia seeds, almond milk, matcha powder, and sweetener (if desired).
2. Cover the bowl and refrigerate for at least 2 hours or overnight.
3. Stir the mixture well before serving, and add toppings like fresh berries or nuts if desired.

3. Blueberry and Walnut Oatmeal Bars:

Ingredients:

- 1 1/2 cups rolled oats
- 1/2 cup whole wheat flour
- 1/4 cup honey or maple syrup
- 1/4 cup coconut oil, melted
- 1/2 cup blueberries
- 1/4 cup walnuts, chopped

Instructions:

1. Preheat the oven to 350°F (175°C) and line a baking dish with parchment paper.

2. In a mixing bowl, combine the oats, flour, honey or maple syrup, and melted coconut oil.

3. Press half of the mixture into the prepared baking dish.

4. Scatter the blueberries and chopped walnuts over the oat mixture.

5. Crumble the remaining oat mixture over the top.

6. Bake for 25-30 minutes or until golden brown.

7. Allow it to cool completely before cutting into bars.

4. Banana and Walnut Smoothie Bowl:
   Ingredients:
   - 2 ripe bananas, frozen
   - 1/2 cup almond milk (or any other milk of your choice)
   - 1 tablespoon almond butter
   - 1 tablespoon honey or maple syrup
   - 1/4 cup walnuts, chopped
   - Optional toppings: sliced bananas, chia seeds, granola

   Instructions:
   1. In a blender, combine the frozen bananas, almond milk, almond butter, and sweetener.
   2. Blend until smooth and creamy.
   3. Pour the smoothie into a bowl and top with chopped walnuts and any other desired toppings.

5. Coconut and Berry Parfait:

Ingredients:

- 1 cup coconut yoghourt

- 1/2 cup mixed berries (such as strawberries, blueberries, and raspberries)

- 1/4 cup granola

- 1 tablespoon honey or maple syrup (optional)

Instructions:

1. In a glass or jar, layer coconut yoghourt, mixed berries, and granola.

2. Repeat the layers until the glass or jar is filled.

3. Drizzle honey or maple syrup on top if desired.

4. Serve immediately or refrigerate until ready to enjoy.

6. Turmeric and Ginger Golden Milk Popsicles:

Ingredients:

- 1 can (13.5 oz) full-fat coconut milk

- 1 teaspoon ground turmeric

- 1/2 teaspoon ground ginger

- 2 tablespoons honey or maple syrup

Instructions:

1. In a blender, combine the coconut milk, turmeric, ginger, and sweetener.

2. Blend until well combined.

3. Pour the mixture into popsicle moulds.

4. Freeze for at least 4 hours or until completely solid.

5. Remove the popsicles from the moulds and enjoy.

7. Avocado Chocolate Mousse:

Ingredients:

- 2 ripe avocados

- 1/4 cup unsweetened cocoa powder

- 1/4 cup honey or maple syrup

- 1 teaspoon vanilla extract

Instructions:

1. Scoop out the flesh of the avocados and place them in a blender or food processor.

2. Add the cocoa powder, honey or maple syrup, and vanilla extract.

3. Blend until smooth and creamy.

4. Spoon the mousse into serving dishes and refrigerate for at least 1 hour before serving.

8. Walnut and Date Energy Balls:

Ingredients:

- 1 cup walnuts

- 1 cup dates, pitted

- 2 tablespoons unsweetened cocoa powder

- 1 tablespoon honey or maple syrup

- 1/4 teaspoon vanilla extract

- Desiccated coconut for rolling (optional)

Instructions:

1. In a food processor, blend the walnuts until finely ground.

2. Add the dates, cocoa powder, honey or maple syrup, and vanilla extract to the food processor.

3. Blend until the mixture comes together and forms a sticky dough.

4. Roll the mixture into small balls and coat them in desiccated coconut if desired.

5. Refrigerate for at least 30 minutes before enjoying.

9. Lemon and Blueberry Yogurt Parfait:

Ingredients:

- 1 cup Greek yoghourt
- 1 tablespoon lemon zest
- 1 tablespoon lemon juice
- 1 tablespoon honey or maple syrup
- 1/2 cup blueberries
- 1/4 cup granola

Instructions:

1. In a bowl, mix the Greek yoghourt, lemon zest, lemon juice, and sweetener.

2. In a glass or jar, layer the yoghourt mixture, blueberries, and granola.

3. Repeat the layers until the glass or jar is filled.

4. Serve immediately or refrigerate until ready to enjoy.

10. Raspberry and Almond Chia Seed Pudding:
Ingredients:
- 1/4 cup chia seeds
- 1 cup almond milk (or any other milk of your choice)
- 1/2 teaspoon almond extract
- 1 tablespoon honey or maple syrup
- 1/2 cup fresh raspberries

Instructions:
1. In a bowl, whisk together the chia seeds, almond milk, almond extract, and sweetener.

2. Cover the bowl and refrigerate for at least 2 hours or overnight.

3. Stir the mixture well before serving.

4. Top with fresh raspberries and enjoy.

Mind-Boosting Dark Chocolate Creations

1. Dark Chocolate Covered Strawberries:

Ingredients:

- Fresh strawberries

- Dark chocolate chips

Instructions:

1. Wash and dry the strawberries.

2. Melt the dark chocolate chips in a microwave-safe bowl.

3. Dip each strawberry into the melted chocolate, coating it completely.

4. Place the strawberries on a parchment-lined baking sheet and let them cool until the chocolate hardens.

5. Enjoy!

2. Dark Chocolate and Almond Energy Balls:

Ingredients:
- 1 cup almonds
- 1 cup dates, pitted
- 2 tablespoons unsweetened cocoa powder
- 1 tablespoon almond butter
- 1 tablespoon honey or maple syrup
- 1/4 teaspoon vanilla extract

Instructions:
1. In a food processor, blend the almonds until finely ground.
2. Add the dates, cocoa powder, almond butter, honey or maple syrup, and vanilla extract.
3. Pulse until the mixture comes together and forms a sticky dough.
4. Roll the mixture into small balls and refrigerate for at least 30 minutes before enjoying.

3. Dark Chocolate Avocado Mousse:
Ingredients:
- 2 ripe avocados

- 1/4 cup unsweetened cocoa powder
- 1/4 cup honey or maple syrup
- 1 teaspoon vanilla extract

Instructions:

1. Scoop out the flesh of the avocados and place them in a blender or food processor.

2. Add the cocoa powder, honey or maple syrup, and vanilla extract.

3. Blend until smooth and creamy.

4. Spoon the mousse into serving dishes and refrigerate for at least 1 hour before serving.

4. Dark Chocolate Trail Mix Bark:

Ingredients:

- 8 ounces dark chocolate, chopped
- 1/2 cup mixed nuts (such as almonds, cashews, and walnuts)
- 1/4 cup dried fruit (such as cranberries, raisins, or cherries)
- 1/4 cup unsweetened shredded coconut

Instructions:

1. Melt the dark chocolate in a microwave-safe bowl or using a double boiler.

2. Stir in the mixed nuts, dried fruit, and shredded coconut.

3. Pour the mixture onto a parchment-lined baking sheet and spread it evenly.

4. Allow it to cool and harden in the refrigerator for about 1 hour.

5. Once hardened, break the bark into smaller pieces and enjoy.

5. Dark Chocolate and Raspberry Chia Pudding:
Ingredients:
- 2 tablespoons chia seeds
- 1 cup almond milk (or any other milk of your choice)
- 1 tablespoon unsweetened cocoa powder
- 1 tablespoon honey or maple syrup
- 1/4 cup fresh raspberries

Instructions:

1. In a bowl, whisk together the chia seeds, almond milk, cocoa powder, and sweetener.

2. Cover the bowl and refrigerate for at least 2 hours or overnight.

3. Stir the mixture well before serving.

4. Top with fresh raspberries and enjoy.

6. Dark Chocolate and Peanut Butter Smoothie:

Ingredients:

- 1 ripe banana

- 1 cup almond milk (or any other milk of your choice)

- 2 tablespoons unsweetened cocoa powder

- 1 tablespoon peanut butter

- 1 tablespoon honey or maple syrup

Instructions:

1. In a blender, combine the ripe banana, almond milk, cocoa powder, peanut butter, and sweetener.

2. Blend until smooth and creamy.

3. Pour into a glass and enjoy.

7. Dark Chocolate and Hazelnut Spread:

Ingredients:

- 1 cup hazelnuts

- 1/4 cup unsweetened cocoa powder

- 2 tablespoons honey or maple syrup

- 1/4 teaspoon vanilla extract

- Pinch of salt

Instructions:

1. Preheat the oven to 350°F (175°C).

2. Spread the hazelnuts on a baking sheet and roast them for about 10-12 minutes until fragrant.

3. Allow the hazelnuts to cool slightly, then transfer them to a clean kitchen towel and rub to remove the skins.

4. In a food processor, blend the hazelnuts until finely ground.

5. Add the cocoa powder, honey or maple syrup, vanilla extract, and salt.

6. Process until smooth and creamy.

7. Transfer the spread to a jar and refrigerate until ready to use.

8. Dark Chocolate and Coconut Chia Seed Pudding:

Ingredients:

- 2 tablespoons chia seeds

- 1 cup coconut milk

- 1 tablespoon unsweetened cocoa powder

- 1 tablespoon honey or maple syrup

- 2 tablespoons shredded coconut

Instructions:

1. In a bowl, whisk together the chia seeds, coconut milk, cocoa powder, and sweetener.

2. Cover the bowl and refrigerate for at least 2 hours or overnight.

3. Stir the mixture well before serving.

4. Top with shredded coconut and enjoy.

9. Dark Chocolate and Blueberry Smoothie Bowl:
Ingredients:
- 2 ripe bananas, frozen
- 1/2 cup almond milk (or any other milk of your choice)
- 1 tablespoon unsweetened cocoa powder
- 1/4 cup dark chocolate chips
- 1/2 cup fresh blueberries
- Optional toppings: sliced banana, granola, chia seeds

Instructions:
1. In a blender, combine the frozen bananas, almond milk, cocoa powder, and dark chocolate chips.
2. Blend until smooth and creamy.
3. Pour the smoothie into a bowl and top with fresh blueberries and any other desired toppings.

10. Dark Chocolate and Matcha Green Tea Truffles:

Ingredients:

- 8 ounces dark chocolate, chopped

- 1/2 cup heavy cream

- 1 tablespoon matcha green tea powder

- Cocoa powder or matcha powder for dusting

Instructions:

1. In a saucepan, heat the heavy cream until it just starts to simmer.

2. Remove from heat and add the chopped dark chocolate and matcha powder.

3. Stir until the chocolate is completely melted and the mixture is smooth.

4. Pour the mixture into a shallow dish and refrigerate for at least 2 hours or until firm.

5. Once firm, use a spoon or a small cookie scoop to form truffle balls.

6. Roll the truffles in cocoa powder or matcha powder to coat.

7. Store in the refrigerator until ready to enjoy.

Fruity Delights to Ignite Your Brain

1. Berry Blast Smoothie:

Ingredients:

- 1 cup mixed berries (strawberries, blueberries, raspberries)

- 1 banana

- 1 cup almond milk (or any other milk of your choice)

- 1 tablespoon honey or maple syrup

- 1 tablespoon chia seeds (optional)

Instructions:

1. In a blender, combine the mixed berries, banana, almond milk, honey or maple syrup, and chia seeds (if using).

2. Blend until smooth and creamy.

3. Pour into a glass and enjoy.

2. Citrus Salad:

Ingredients:
- 2 oranges, peeled and segmented
- 1 grapefruit, peeled and segmented
- 1 tablespoon honey or maple syrup
- Fresh mint leaves for garnish

Instructions:
1. In a bowl, combine the orange and grapefruit segments.
2. Drizzle with honey or maple syrup.
3. Garnish with fresh mint leaves.
4. Toss gently to combine.
5. Serve chilled.

3. Tropical Fruit Parfait:
Ingredients:
- 1 cup diced pineapple
- 1 cup diced mango
- 1 cup Greek yoghourt
- 1/4 cup granola
- 1 tablespoon shredded coconut

Instructions:

1. In a glass or bowl, layer the diced pineapple, diced mango, and Greek yoghourt.

2. Sprinkle it with granola and shredded coconut.

3. Repeat the layers.

4. Finish with a sprinkle of granola and shredded coconut.

5. Serve chilled.

4. Kiwi and Banana Nice Cream:

Ingredients:

- 2 ripe bananas, frozen

- 2 kiwis, peeled and sliced

- 1 tablespoon honey or maple syrup

- Fresh mint leaves for garnish

Instructions:

1. In a blender or food processor, blend the frozen bananas, kiwis, and honey or maple syrup until smooth and creamy.

2. Transfer the mixture into a bowl.

3. Garnish with fresh mint leaves.

4. Serve immediately.

5. Watermelon and Feta Salad:
Ingredients:
   - 2 cups cubed watermelon
   - 1/2 cup crumbled feta cheese
   - 1/4 cup fresh mint leaves, torn
   - 1 tablespoon balsamic glaze

Instructions:
   1. In a bowl, combine the cubed watermelon, crumbled feta cheese, and torn mint leaves.

   2. Drizzle with balsamic glaze.

   3. Toss gently to combine.

   4. Serve chilled.

6. Blueberry and Almond Overnight Oats:
Ingredients:
   - 1/2 cup rolled oats

- 1/2 cup almond milk (or any other milk of your choice)
  - 1/4 cup Greek yoghourt
  - 1/4 cup fresh blueberries
  - 1 tablespoon almond butter
  - 1 tablespoon honey or maple syrup

Instructions:

1. In a jar or container, combine the rolled oats, almond milk, Greek yoghourt, fresh blueberries, almond butter, and honey or maple syrup.

2. Stir well to combine.

3. Cover and refrigerate overnight.

4. In the morning, give it a good stir and enjoy.

7. Mango and Coconut Chia Pudding:

Ingredients:
  - 2 tablespoons chia seeds
  - 1 cup coconut milk
  - 1 ripe mango, diced
  - 1 tablespoon honey or maple syrup

- Shredded coconut for garnish

Instructions:

1. In a bowl, whisk together the chia seeds, coconut milk, diced mango, and honey or maple syrup.

2. Cover the bowl and refrigerate for at least 2 hours or overnight.

3. Stir the mixture well before serving.

4. Garnish with shredded coconut.

5. Enjoy chilled.

8. Pineapple and Ginger Infused Water:
Ingredients:
- 1/2 cup diced pineapple
- 1-inch piece of fresh ginger, sliced
- 4 cups water
- Ice cubes

Instructions:

1. In a pitcher, combine the diced pineapple, sliced ginger, and water.

2. Let it infuse in the refrigerator for at least 1 hour.

3. Serve over ice cubes.

9. Raspberry and Dark Chocolate Yogurt Bark:

Ingredients:

- 1 cup Greek yoghourt

- 1/4 cup fresh raspberries

- 2 tablespoons dark chocolate chips

Instructions:

1. Line a baking sheet with parchment paper.

2. Spread the Greek yoghourt evenly on the parchment paper.

3. Scatter the fresh raspberries and dark chocolate chips on top.

4. Place the baking sheet in the freezer for at least 2 hours or until firm.

5. Once firm, break the bark into smaller pieces and enjoy.

10. Strawberry and Spinach Salad:
   Ingredients:
   - 2 cups baby spinach
   - 1 cup sliced strawberries
   - 1/4 cup crumbled goat cheese
   - 1/4 cup sliced almonds
   - Balsamic vinaigrette dressing

Instructions:
   1. In a bowl, combine the baby spinach, sliced strawberries, crumbled goat cheese, and sliced almonds.
   2. Drizzle with balsamic vinaigrette dressing.
   3. Toss gently to combine.
   4. Serve chilled.

Chapter 7: Beverages for Cognitive Refreshment

1. Matcha Green Tea Latte:

Ingredients:

- 1 teaspoon matcha green tea powder

- 1 cup almond milk (or any milk of your choice)

- 1 tablespoon honey (optional)

Instructions:

1. In a small saucepan, heat almond milk over medium heat until hot but not boiling.

2. In a cup, whisk together matcha green tea powder and a small amount of hot almond milk to form a smooth paste.

3. Gradually whisk in the remaining almond milk.

4. Add honey if desired, and stir until well combined.

5. Serve hot.

2. Turmeric Golden Milk:

Ingredients:
- 1 cup almond milk (or any milk of your choice)
- 1/2 teaspoon turmeric powder
- 1/4 teaspoon cinnamon powder
- 1/4 teaspoon ginger powder
- 1 tablespoon honey (optional)

Instructions:

1. In a small saucepan, heat almond milk over medium heat until hot but not boiling.

2. Add turmeric powder, cinnamon powder, ginger powder, and honey (if desired).

3. Stir well until all ingredients are dissolved.

4. Pour into a cup and serve hot.

3. Berry Blast Smoothie:

Ingredients:
- 1 cup mixed berries (such as blueberries, strawberries, and raspberries)
- 1 banana
- 1 cup almond milk (or any milk of your choice)

- 1 tablespoon honey (optional)

- 1 tablespoon chia seeds (optional)

Instructions:

1. In a blender, combine mixed berries, banana, almond milk, and honey (if desired).

2. Blend until smooth and creamy.

3. If desired, stir in chia seeds for added texture and nutrients.

4. Pour into a glass and serve chilled.

4. Coconut Water with Lime:

Ingredients:

- 1 cup coconut water

- Juice of 1 lime

- Fresh mint leaves for garnish (optional)

Instructions:

1. In a glass, mix together coconut water and lime juice.

2. Stir well to combine.

3. Garnish with fresh mint leaves if desired.

4. Serve chilled.

5. Fresh Ginger and Lemon Tea:
Ingredients:
- 1-inch piece of fresh ginger, peeled and sliced
- Juice of 1 lemon
- 1 tablespoon honey (optional)

Instructions:
1. In a small saucepan, bring 2 cups of water to a boil.

2. Add ginger slices and reduce heat to low.

3. Let the ginger simmer for 5 minutes.

4. Remove from heat and strain the ginger-infused water into a cup.

5. Add lemon juice and honey (if desired).

6. Stir until well combined.

7. Serve hot.

6. Beetroot and Carrot Juice:

Ingredients:

- 1 medium-sized beetroot, peeled and chopped

- 2 medium-sized carrots, peeled and chopped

- Juice of 1 orange

- 1 tablespoon lemon juice

Instructions:

1. In a juicer, process beetroot and carrots to extract the juice.

2. Pour the juice into a glass.

3. Add orange juice and lemon juice.

4. Stir well to combine.

5. Serve chilled.

7. Peppermint and Green Tea Infusion:

Ingredients:

- 1 green tea bag

- 1 peppermint tea bag

- 2 cups hot water

- Honey or stevia (optional)

Instructions:

1. Place a green tea bag and peppermint tea bag in a teapot or cup.

2. Pour hot water over the tea bags.

3. Let the tea steep for 5-7 minutes.

4. Remove the tea bags and add honey or stevia if desired.

5. Stir until the sweetener is dissolved.

6. Serve hot.

8. Fresh Orange and Ginger Smoothie:

Ingredients:

- 2 oranges, peeled and segmented

- 1-inch piece of fresh ginger, peeled and grated

- 1 cup almond milk (or any milk of your choice)

- 1 tablespoon honey (optional)

- Ice cubes

Instructions:

1. In a blender, combine orange segments, grated ginger, almond milk, honey (if desired), and ice cubes.

2. Blend until smooth and frothy.

3. Pour into a glass and serve chilled.

9. Cucumber and Mint Infused Water:

Ingredients:

- 1/2 cucumber, sliced

- A handful of fresh mint leaves

- 4 cups water

- Ice cubes

Instructions:

1. In a pitcher, combine cucumber slices, mint leaves, and water.

2. Stir well to combine.

3. Refrigerate for at least 2 hours to allow the flavours to infuse.

4. Add ice cubes before serving.

5. Serve chilled.

10. Iced Green Tea with Lemon:

Ingredients:

- 2 green tea bags

- 4 cups hot water

- Juice of 1 lemon

- 1 tablespoon honey (optional)

- Ice cubes

Instructions:

1. Place green tea bags in a pitcher or jug.

2. Pour hot water over the tea bags.

3. Let the tea steep for 5-7 minutes.

4. Remove the tea bags and add lemon juice and honey (if desired).

5. Stir until well combined.

6. Refrigerate for at least 2 hours to cool.

7. Add ice cubes before serving.

8. Serve chilled.

Brain-Fueling Smoothies and Juices

1. Blueberry Brain Boost Smoothie:

Ingredients:

- 1 cup blueberries

- 1 banana

- 1 cup almond milk (or any milk of your choice)

- 1 tablespoon almond butter

- 1 tablespoon chia seeds

Instructions:

1. In a blender, combine blueberries, banana, almond milk, almond butter, and chia seeds.

2. Blend until smooth and creamy.

3. Pour into a glass and serve chilled.

2. Spinach and Avocado Power Juice:

Ingredients:

- 2 cups spinach

- 1 ripe avocado

- 1 green apple

- Juice of 1 lemon

- 1 cup coconut water

Instructions:

1. In a juicer, process spinach, avocado, green apple, and lemon juice to extract the juice.

2. Pour the juice into a glass.

3. Add coconut water and stir well to combine.

4. Serve chilled.

3. Kale and Pineapple Brain Booster Smoothie:

Ingredients:

- 2 cups kale leaves

- 1 cup pineapple chunks

- 1 banana

- 1 cup coconut water

- 1 tablespoon flax seeds

Instructions:

1. In a blender, combine kale leaves, pineapple chunks, banana, coconut water, and flaxseeds.

2. Blend until smooth and creamy.

3. Pour into a glass and serve chilled.

4. Beetroot and Berry Brain Elixir:
   Ingredients:
   - 1 small beetroot, peeled and chopped
     - 1 cup mixed berries (such as blueberries, strawberries, and raspberries)
   - 1 tablespoon honey
   - 1 cup water

   Instructions:
   1. In a blender, combine beetroot, mixed berries, honey, and water.
   2. Blend until smooth and well combined.
   3. Pour into a glass and serve chilled.

5. Mango and Coconut Brain Smoothie:
   Ingredients:
   - 1 ripe mango, peeled and chopped
   - 1 cup coconut milk
   - 1 tablespoon hemp seeds
   - 1 tablespoon honey (optional)

Instructions:

1. In a blender, combine mango, coconut milk, hemp seeds, and honey (if desired).

2. Blend until smooth and creamy.

3. Pour into a glass and serve chilled.

6. Carrot and Ginger Brain Booster Juice:

Ingredients:

- 3 medium-sized carrots, peeled and chopped
- 1-inch piece of fresh ginger, peeled and grated
- Juice of 1 orange
- 1 tablespoon turmeric powder
- 1 cup water

Instructions:

1. In a juicer, process carrots and ginger to extract the juice.

2. Pour the juice into a glass.

3. Add orange juice, turmeric powder, and water.

4. Stir well to combine.

5. Serve chilled.

7. Peanut Butter and Banana Brain Smoothie:
Ingredients:
- 1 banana
- 2 tablespoons peanut butter
- 1 cup almond milk (or any milk of your choice)
- 1 tablespoon honey (optional)
- 1 tablespoon cocoa powder (optional)

Instructions:
1. In a blender, combine banana, peanut butter, almond milk, honey (if desired), and cocoa powder (if desired).
2. Blend until smooth and creamy.
3. Pour into a glass and serve chilled.

8. Green Tea and Berry Brain Refresher:
Ingredients:
- 1 green tea bag

- 1 cup mixed berries (such as blueberries, strawberries, and raspberries)
- Juice of 1 lemon
- 1 cup water
- Ice cubes

Instructions:

1. Steep the green tea bag in hot water for 5 minutes.

2. Remove the tea bag and let the tea cool.

3. In a blender, combine green tea, mixed berries, lemon juice, and water.

4. Blend until smooth and well combined.

5. Add ice cubes and blend again until desired consistency.

6. Pour into a glass and serve chilled.

9. Walnut and Banana Brain Boost Smoothie:
Ingredients:
- 1 banana
- 1/2 cup walnuts

- 1 cup almond milk (or any milk of your choice)

- 1 tablespoon honey (optional)

- 1/2 teaspoon cinnamon powder

Instructions:

1. In a blender, combine banana, walnuts, almond milk, honey (if desired), and cinnamon powder.

2. Blend until smooth and creamy.

3. Pour into a glass and serve chilled.

10. Raspberry and Oat Brain Fuel Smoothie:

Ingredients:

- 1 cup raspberries

- 1/2 cup cooked oats

- 1 cup almond milk (or any milk of your choice)

- 1 tablespoon honey (optional)

- 1 tablespoon almond butter

Instructions:

1. In a blender, combine raspberries, cooked oats, almond milk, honey (if desired), and almond butter.

2. Blend until smooth and creamy.

3. Pour into a glass and serve chilled.

Herbal Teas for Mental Clarity

1. Rosemary and Lemon Balm Tea:

Ingredients:

- 1 tablespoon dried rosemary

- 1 tablespoon dried lemon balm

- 2 cups water

Instructions:

1. In a small pot, bring water to a boil.

2. Add dried rosemary and lemon balm to the boiling water.

3. Reduce heat and let the herbs steep for 10 minutes.

4. Strain the tea into a cup and enjoy.

2. Peppermint and Ginseng Tea:

Ingredients:

- 1 tablespoon dried peppermint leaves

- 1 tablespoon dried ginseng root

- 2 cups water

Instructions:

1. Bring water to a boil in a small pot.

2. Add dried peppermint leaves and ginseng root to the boiling water.

3. Reduce heat and let the herbs steep for 5-7 minutes.

4. Strain the tea into a cup and enjoy.

3. Gotu Kola and Green Tea Blend:

Ingredients:

- 1 tablespoon dried kola leaves

- 1 green tea bag

- 2 cups water

Instructions:

1. Boil water in a small pot.

2. Add dried kola leaves and a green tea bag to the boiling water.

3. Let the herbs steep for 3-5 minutes.

4. Remove the tea bag and strain the tea into a cup.

5. Enjoy the blend of kola and green tea.

4. Sage and Holy Basil Tea:
Ingredients:
- 1 tablespoon dried sage leaves
- 1 tablespoon dried holy basil leaves
- 2 cups water

Instructions:
1. Bring water to a boil in a small pot.

2. Add dried sage leaves and holy basil leaves to the boiling water.

3. Reduce heat and let the herbs steep for 10 minutes.

4. Strain the tea into a cup and enjoy.

5. Lemon Verbena and Chamomile Tea:

Ingredients:

- 1 tablespoon dried lemon verbena leaves

- 1 tablespoon dried chamomile flowers

- 2 cups water

Instructions:

1. Boil water in a small pot.

2. Add dried lemon verbena leaves and chamomile flowers to the boiling water.

3. Let the herbs steep for 5-7 minutes.

4. Strain the tea into a cup and enjoy.

6. Ginkgo Biloba and LemonGrass Tea:

Ingredients:

- 1 tablespoon dried ginkgo biloba leaves

- 1 tablespoon dried lemon grass

- 2 cups water

Instructions:

1. Bring water to a boil in a small pot.

2. Add dried ginkgo biloba leaves and lemon grass to the boiling water.

3. Reduce heat and let the herbs steep for 10 minutes.

4. Strain the tea into a cup and enjoy.

7. Lavender and Passionflower Tea:

Ingredients:

- 1 tablespoon dried lavender flowers
- 1 tablespoon dried passion flower leaves
- 2 cups water

Instructions:

1. Boil water in a small pot.

2. Add dried lavender flowers and passionflower leaves to the boiling water.

3. Let the herbs steep for 5-7 minutes.

4. Strain the tea into a cup and enjoy.

8. Lemon Balm and Chamomile Tea:

Ingredients:

- 1 tablespoon dried lemon balm leaves

- 1 tablespoon dried chamomile flowers

- 2 cups water

Instructions:

1. Bring water to a boil in a small pot.

2. Add dried lemon balm leaves and chamomile flowers to the boiling water.

3. Reduce heat and let the herbs steep for 10 minutes.

4. Strain the tea into a cup and enjoy.

9. Rosehip and Hibiscus Tea:

Ingredients:

- 1 tablespoon dried rosehip

- 1 tablespoon dried hibiscus flowers

- 2 cups water

Instructions:

1. Boil water in a small pot.

2. Add dried rosehip and hibiscus flowers to the boiling water.

3. Let the herbs steep for 5-7 minutes.

4. Strain the tea into a cup and enjoy.

10. Lemon Verbena and Ginger Tea:
Ingredients:
- 1 tablespoon dried lemon verbena leaves
- 1-inch piece of fresh ginger, sliced
- 2 cups water

Instructions:
1. Bring water to a boil in a small pot.

2. Add dried lemon verbena leaves and sliced ginger to the boiling water.

3. Reduce heat and let the herbs steep for 10 minutes.

4. Strain the tea into a cup and enjoy.

Chapter 8: Meal Planning and Tips for a Brain-Healthy Lifestyle

Maintaining a brain-healthy lifestyle is essential for overall well-being and cognitive function. One key aspect of this lifestyle is meal planning, which involves carefully selecting and preparing meals that nourish the brain. Here are some comprehensive tips to help you incorporate brain-healthy foods into your meal plan:

1. Include Omega-3 Fatty Acids: Omega-3 fatty acids are crucial for brain health. Incorporate fatty fish such as salmon, mackerel, and sardines into your diet at least twice a week. If you're vegetarian or vegan, opt for plant-based sources like flaxseeds, chia seeds, and walnuts.

2. Load Up on Antioxidants: Antioxidants help protect the brain from oxidative stress and

inflammation. Include a variety of colourful fruits and vegetables in your meals, such as berries, leafy greens, broccoli, tomatoes, and bell peppers. These are rich in vitamins, minerals, and phytochemicals that support brain health.

3. Choose Whole Grains: Whole grains provide a steady release of energy and contain essential nutrients like fibre, B vitamins, and antioxidants. Opt for whole grain options like brown rice, quinoa, whole wheat bread, and oatmeal. These help maintain stable blood sugar levels and support brain function.

4. Emphasise Healthy Fats: Healthy fats, such as those found in avocados, olive oil, nuts, and seeds, are essential for brain health. They provide a source of energy and support the growth and function of brain cells. Use these fats for cooking, salad dressings, or as toppings for meals.

5. Limit Added Sugars: Excessive sugar consumption can lead to inflammation and negatively impact brain health. Reduce your intake of sugary beverages, processed snacks, and desserts. Instead, satisfy your sweet tooth with naturally sweet fruits or opt for healthier alternatives like stevia or honey in moderation.

6. Stay Hydrated: Dehydration can affect cognitive function and mood. Drink plenty of water throughout the day to stay properly hydrated. You can also include herbal teas or infuse water with slices of fruits like lemon, cucumber, or berries for added flavour.

7. Mindful Eating: Practise mindful eating to fully enjoy and appreciate your meals. Slow down, savour the flavours, and pay attention to your body's hunger and fullness cues. This helps prevent overeating and promotes a healthier relationship with food.

8. Plan and Prep Meals: Set aside time each week for meal planning and preparation. Plan your meals in advance to ensure a balanced and brain-healthy diet. Consider batch cooking or preparing ingredients in advance to save time during busy weekdays.

9. Balance Macronutrients: Include a balance of macronutrients in your meals. Aim for a combination of lean proteins (such as poultry, fish, tofu, or legumes), complex carbohydrates (like whole grains, beans, and starchy vegetables), and healthy fats. This combination provides sustained energy and supports brain function.

10. Reduce Processed Foods: Minimise your consumption of processed foods, which often contain high levels of unhealthy fats, added sugars, and artificial additives. Opt for whole, unprocessed foods whenever possible.

Remember, a brain-healthy lifestyle is not just about what you eat but also includes regular physical exercise, quality sleep, stress management, and cognitive stimulation. By combining these elements, you can optimise your brain health and overall well-being.

Creating Balanced and Nutritious Meal Plans

A balanced and nutritious meal plan is crucial for maintaining optimal health and well-being. It ensures that your body receives all the necessary nutrients, vitamins, and minerals it needs to function properly. Here are some comprehensive tips to help you create a balanced and nutritious meal plan:

1. Determine Your Caloric Needs: Start by calculating your daily caloric needs based on factors such as age, gender, weight, activity level, and goals (e.g., weight loss, maintenance, or muscle gain).

This will provide a baseline for planning your meals.

2. Include a Variety of Food Groups: A balanced meal plan should incorporate foods from all the major food groups, including fruits, vegetables, whole grains, lean proteins, and healthy fats. This ensures that you obtain a wide range of nutrients and phytochemicals.

3. Portion Control: Pay attention to portion sizes to avoid overeating. Use measuring cups, a food scale, or visual cues to ensure you're consuming appropriate portions of each food group. This helps maintain a healthy weight and prevents excessive calorie intake.

4. Fill Half Your Plate with Fruits and Vegetables: Aim to fill at least half of your plate with a colourful variety of fruits and vegetables. They are rich in fibre, vitamins, minerals, and antioxidants.

Include both raw and cooked options to maximise nutrient intake.

5. Choose Whole Grains: Opt for whole grains such as brown rice, quinoa, whole wheat bread, oats, and whole grain pasta. They are higher in fibre and nutrients compared to refined grains, which have been stripped of their bran and germ.

6. Incorporate Lean Proteins: Include lean sources of protein in your meal plan, such as skinless poultry, fish, tofu, legumes, lentils, and low-fat dairy products. These provide essential amino acids for muscle repair and growth.

7. Include Healthy Fats: Incorporate sources of healthy fats like avocados, nuts, seeds, olive oil, and fatty fish. These fats are important for brain function, hormone production, and nutrient absorption. However, be mindful of portion sizes as fats are calorie-dense.

8. Limit Added Sugars and Processed Foods: Minimise your intake of added sugars found in sugary drinks, desserts, and processed snacks. Instead, opt for natural sweeteners like fruits or small amounts of honey or maple syrup. Reduce your consumption of processed foods that are often high in unhealthy fats, sodium, and artificial additives.

9. Plan Meals in Advance: Take time to plan your meals in advance to ensure a balanced and nutritious diet. Create a weekly meal plan and make a shopping list accordingly. This helps prevent impulsive food choices and ensures you have all the ingredients needed for healthy meals.

10. Prepare Meals at Home: Cooking meals at home allows you to have control over the ingredients and cooking methods used. This helps reduce the consumption of unhealthy additives and

excessive sodium. Experiment with new recipes and cooking techniques to keep your meals interesting and enjoyable.

11. Stay Hydrated: Don't forget to include adequate hydration in your meal plan. Drink plenty of water throughout the day and limit sugary beverages. Opt for herbal teas or infused water for added flavour and hydration.

12. Listen to Your Body: Pay attention to your body's hunger and fullness cues. Eat when you're hungry and stop when you're comfortably full. Avoid restrictive diets or skipping meals, as this can lead to nutrient deficiencies and unhealthy eating patterns.

Remember, creating a balanced and nutritious meal plan is a personalised process. It's important to consider individual dietary needs, preferences, and any specific health conditions. Consulting with a registered dietitian can provide personalised guidance and support in creating a meal plan that suits your unique needs and goals.

Smart Grocery Shopping for Brain-Boosting Ingredients

The food we consume plays a critical role in brain health and function. By incorporating brain-boosting ingredients into our diets, we can support cognitive function, improve memory, and enhance overall brain health. Here are some comprehensive tips for smart grocery shopping to ensure you're selecting the right ingredients to nourish your brain:

1. Prioritise Fresh Fruits and Vegetables: Fill your shopping cart with a variety of colourful fruits and vegetables. These are rich in antioxidants, vitamins, and minerals that support brain health. Look for leafy greens like spinach and kale, berries such as

blueberries and strawberries, and cruciferous vegetables like broccoli and cauliflower.

2. Include Omega-3 Fatty Acids: Omega-3 fatty acids, particularly DHA, are essential for brain health. Incorporate fatty fish like salmon, sardines, and mackerel into your diet. If you're vegetarian or vegan, opt for plant-based sources of omega-3s like flaxseeds, chia seeds, walnuts, and hemp seeds.

3. Choose Whole Grains: Whole grains provide a steady supply of glucose to the brain, which is its main source of energy. Opt for whole grain options like brown rice, quinoa, oats, whole wheat bread, and whole grain pasta. These are rich in fibre, vitamins, and minerals that support brain function.

4. Include Healthy Fats: Healthy fats are essential for brain health, as they support the structure and function of brain cells. Look for sources of monounsaturated fats like avocados, olive oil, and

nuts. Incorporate small amounts of saturated fats from sources like coconut oil and grass-fed butter. Avoid trans fats found in processed and fried foods, as they can have detrimental effects on brain health.

5. Include Nuts and Seeds: Nuts and seeds are packed with nutrients that support brain health. Almonds, walnuts, cashews, and sunflower seeds are rich in vitamin E, which has been linked to improved cognitive function. Additionally, they provide healthy fats, fibre, and antioxidants.

6. Incorporate Beans and Legumes: Beans and legumes are excellent sources of plant-based protein, fibre, and complex carbohydrates. They have a low glycemic index, which means they release glucose into the bloodstream slowly, providing a steady source of energy for the brain. Include options like lentils, chickpeas, black beans, and kidney beans in your shopping list.

7. Look for Dark Chocolate: Dark chocolate with a high cocoa content (70% or more) is rich in antioxidants and flavonoids that can improve cognitive function. Look for dark chocolate without added sugars or artificial additives.

8. Include Herbs and Spices: Certain herbs and spices have been shown to have brain-boosting properties. Turmeric, for example, contains curcumin, which has anti-inflammatory and antioxidant effects. Other brain-boosting herbs and spices include rosemary, sage, cinnamon, and ginger.

9. Read Labels Carefully: When purchasing packaged foods, read the labels carefully to ensure they contain brain-healthy ingredients. Avoid products that are high in added sugars, artificial additives, and unhealthy fats. Look for products that are minimally processed and made with whole food ingredients.

10. Stay Hydrated: Proper hydration is essential for optimal brain function. Drink plenty of water throughout the day and limit sugary beverages. If you're looking for a brain-boosting beverage, consider green tea, which contains antioxidants and caffeine that can enhance cognitive function.

11. Plan Ahead: Before heading to the grocery store, plan your meals for the week and create a shopping list. This will help you stay focused and avoid impulsive purchases of unhealthy foods. Include brain-boosting ingredients in your meal plan and ensure you have everything you need to prepare nutritious meals.

Remember, a healthy diet is just one aspect of maintaining brain health. Regular exercise, adequate sleep, stress management, and mental stimulation are also important for optimal brain function. By incorporating brain-boosting ingredients into your diet and adopting a holistic approach to brain health, you can support cognitive function and enhance overall well-being.

As we come to the end of this book, it is my hope that you have gained valuable insights and knowledge on creating balanced and nutritious meal plans, as well as the importance of smart grocery shopping for brain-boosting ingredients. Throughout this journey, we have explored the vital role that food plays in nourishing our bodies and minds.

By understanding the power of a well-planned meal, you have discovered how to provide your body with the necessary nutrients it needs to thrive. From incorporating a variety of fruits and vegetables to choosing whole grains and lean proteins, you have learned how to create balanced and nutritious meals that support optimal health.

Moreover, you have delved into the world of brain-boosting ingredients, understanding how certain foods can enhance cognitive function and promote brain health. By prioritising fresh fruits and vegetables, including omega-3 fatty acids, and embracing healthy fats, you have unlocked the potential to support your brain's vitality and overall well-being.

But this journey does not end here. The knowledge you have gained must now be put into action. It is time to take what you have learned and apply it to your daily life. Embrace the power of smart grocery shopping, filling your cart with wholesome ingredients that will nourish your body and mind.

Remember, creating a balanced and nutritious meal plan is a personal journey. It requires understanding your own unique needs, preferences, and goals. Listen to your body, pay attention to its signals, and make choices that align with your health and well-being.

As you embark on this new chapter of your life, I encourage you to continue exploring the world of healthy eating. Seek out new recipes, experiment with different ingredients, and never stop learning. Embrace the joy of cooking and the satisfaction that comes from nourishing yourself and those around you.

In closing, I want to remind you that a healthy mind and body are interconnected. By fueling your body with nutritious foods, you are not only supporting physical health but also nurturing your brain and promoting mental well-being. Embrace the power of food as a tool for self-care and self-love.

Thank you for joining me on this journey of creating balanced and nutritious meal plans and embracing smart grocery shopping for brain-boosting ingredients. May your path be filled with delicious meals, vibrant health, and a deep sense of fulfilment. Here's to a life well-nourished, both inside and out.